T0210215

Inheritance in Contemporary America

Inheritance in Contemporary America

The Social Dimensions of Giving across Generations

JACQUELINE L. ANGEL

Professor,
LBJ School of Public Affairs
and Department of Sociology,
The University of Texas at Austin

The Johns Hopkins University Press
Baltimore

© 2008 The Johns Hopkins University Press
All rights reserved. Published 2008
Printed in the United States of America on acid-free paper
2 4 6 8 9 7 5 3 1

The Johns Hopkins University Press
2715 North Charles Street
Baltimore, Maryland 21218-4363
www.press.jhu.edu

Library of Congress Cataloging-in-Publication Data
Angel, Jacqueline Lowe.
Inheritance in contemporary America : the social dimensions of giving across
generations / Jacqueline L. Angel.
p. cm.
Includes bibliographical references and index.
ISBN-13: 978-0-8018-8763-5 (hardcover : alk. paper)
ISBN-10: 0-8018-8763-1 (hardcover : alk. paper)
1. Inheritance and succession—United States. 2. Wealth—United States.
3. Inheritance and transfer tax—United States. 4. Estate planning—United States.
5. Older people—Family relationships—United States. 6. Older people—Care—
United States. 7. Older people—Health and hygiene—United States. I. Title.
HB715.A55 2008
306.3—dc22
2007027880

A catalog record for this book is available from the British Library.

Special discounts are available for bulk purchases of this book. For more information,
please contact Special Sales at 410-516-6936 or specialsales@press.jhu.edu.

The Johns Hopkins University Press uses environmentally friendly book materials,
including recycled text paper that is composed of at least 30 percent post-consumer
waste, whenever possible. All of our book papers are acid-free, and our jackets and
covers are printed on paper with recycled content.

To my beloved husband, Ron,
who has given me so much in my life
and for whom I am enormously grateful

Contents

Preface

I became interested in contemporary inheritance practices while doing research for a book that looked at elderly people and their relationship to their families. In the course of that research, I made the startling discovery that the health of our aging population is inextricably linked to wealth. This fact presents new and important economic, legal, and emotional challenges for the American family. Surprisingly, the topic had largely gone unaddressed by policy makers for decades. Consequently, I have chosen to use a wide sociological lens to better understand the social dimensions and implications of intergenerational transfers, bequests, and inheritance in the United States.

Chapter 1 describes how the transfer of wealth between generations is changing in every regard, thus giving rise to a new social contract in which family will increasingly play a larger role in minimizing risks in later life. A background of U.S. inheritance laws and attitudes from colonial to modern times is given in Chapter 2, which describes some pivotal focal events that underlie inheritance practices today. Chapter 3 examines intergenerational exchanges and wealth transfers from a cross-national perspective. I compare and contrast the current institutional arrangements of pension programs in the United States with those in other industrialized nations, including Sweden, France, and Italy, that are also undergoing dramatic demographic change and challenges in caring for their elderly citizens. The comparison of the old-age welfare state in Europe and the United States helps to further place the topic in context and illuminate the goal of creating policies designed to influence individual-level wealth accumulation.

In Chapter 4, I examine the massive differences among and within families regarding the extent of wealth and inter vivos transfers for college education, home mortgages, and other purposes. I summarize an abundance of statistical data based on nationwide household surveys of ethnically diverse families. The analyses shed light on the variation in gift giving and inheritance patterns across the life cycle. The focus of Chapter 4 is the generational differences between two cohorts, born from 1946 to 1964 (Baby Boom Generation) and those who grew up during the Depression era (Silent Generation). The lifelong shared experiences and events associated with each birth cohort have been found to influence attitudes toward retirement income security (Torres-Gil, 1992). I also look at gift-giving patterns for these different age groups across the economic spectrum, including people of non-Latino white, African American, Asian, and Mexican ancestry.

In Chapter 5, I use both biographical narratives and anecdotal evidence to explore the role of material exchanges in defining the moral ties between generations as they relate to gender, race, class, ethnicity, and religious affiliation. In so doing, I depart from traditional social scientific approaches to collecting data, relying instead on in-depth interviews of intergenerational transfers from the perspective of low-income families to upper-class men and women actively involved in faith-based organizations in Austin, Texas. The case study material reveals what is involved in the decision-making processes and helps to illustrate the generalizations drawn from the surveys.

Chapter 6 fleshes out the concept of contemporary inheritance practices by thinking about how wealth practices have changed over time. The chapter draws on nonquantitative data about patterns of material exchanges and the symbolic aspects of the meaning attached to gift giving from the perspective both of the parent and the adult child. The chapter highlights the centrality of "family ideology" concerning who owes what to whom and expectations regarding reciprocity gifts and bequests. Finally, the chapter specifically addresses filial expectations concerning who should give what to whom in adult child–parent relationships and how feelings of obligation may change as individuals age.

In Chapter 7, I discuss the legal and state institutions influencing the process by which older adults make decisions about gift giving. Extended life spans make estate transfers a lifelong process rather than something that occurs only upon a parent's death. Today, the considerable costs of educating a child and providing a start in life can eat up what in earlier times might eventually have been received as an inheritance. There is a raging public debate on the roles of family, the market, and government in providing care to a loved one. A section focusing on the heart of the debate examines the financial burden of family caregiving. This chapter highlights the complex ethical issues that arise in trying to apply current policies related to the fair distribution of income and wealth across generations. In addition to examining the influence of elder attorneys on the decision-making process about gifting, I investigate the role of interest groups who act on behalf of the elderly population. The research provides empirical evidence on how interest groups such as AARP may interact with the family, the state, and individuals to influence ultimate financial behavior. The end of Chapter 7 summarizes the major social policy issues relating to inter vivos transfers, estate taxes, and inheritance taxes, and their consequences for the distribution of wealth and income.

Chapter 8 documents how political economics coupled with family ideology ultimately determine financial behavior during people's later life. Policy recommendations are offered on how government can buttress the tie between parents and children. The chapter reviews past, current, and anticipated legislation and regulations of intergenerational policies, with special emphasis on how they relate to the costs of paying for old-age welfare programs. Specific laws include federal entitlements and state government practices of estate and inheritance taxation, gift income credit, guardianship laws, Medicaid spend-down (and asset transfer), and the 1993 Omnibus Budget Reconciliation Act (OBRA) Medicaid Estate Recovery programs. This section also assesses how current estate and gift tax laws exacerbate social inequality in the United States.

Finally, I devote the last chapter to a consideration of the importance of the different generational perspectives on intrafamilial income transfers. Toward that end, Chapter 9 synthesizes the major findings, providing a summary and overview of theoretical explanations of late-life gift-giving behavior. In addition, the chapter considers a future research agenda that examines the policy implications of gift giving and wealth transmission trends for generations to come. Lawmakers of all stripes are trying to gauge the costs of family fortunes and lack of wealth on "the state" as social welfare policies and programs profoundly alter the lives of nearly every American, including the young, workers, and persons entering retirement years.

Inheritance in Contemporary America

CHAPTER ONE

The Story of Inheritance

Intergenerational Giving in Aging America

Wealth is the ability to fully experience life.
—*Henry David Thoreau (1817–1862)*

Inheritance takes many forms in our society. Yet, no matter how different we are from each other, to all of us inheritance means passing something of value— wisdom, property, cash—from one generation to a later one. How do our nation's social, demographic, and economic changes affect the concept and practice of a legacy transfer or inheritance? How have our collective and individual experiences influenced our attitudes about inheritance? How do we determine who is worthy of an inheritance?

As the title of this chapter suggests, the questions in this book cover the subject of gift giving, intergenerational transfers, and bequests in a rapidly aging society. What makes this book unusual is that it is largely focused on the emotional and moral implications of wealth transmission and gift-giving behavior from a sociologist's point of view. Also distinctive is its emphasis on contextualizing social aspects of the meaning of gift giving and bequests using a life-course framework. During this investigation of the noneconomic dimension of inheritance, which is largely uncharted territory in the social sciences, it should become clear why this topic deserves serious attention.

The story of inheritance is an intriguing one. Besides kinship and affection, families are defined by material exchanges. Family members have a unique claim on one another's time and wealth, and such exchanges between family members are governed by a different set of rules from those governing exchanges between nonkin. Legally, of course, the "contractual" obligation of a parent to care for the child *is* enforceable: the state can take the child away and assume the child's care if the parent fails to fulfill that part of the parent-child "contract." Under normal circumstances, however, a contract between a parent and a child is not enforced, by virtue of the nature of the bond between them. For instance, would a parent actually take a child to court for nonpayment of a debt? Such behavior would strike most of us as shocking, and the fact is that most parents would never dream of taking things so far.

Gifts from parents to children, at least to some degree, represent early estate transfers. Such exchanges can clearly enhance a young adult's life chances, especially when they are used for education, and they can give great satisfaction to parents. When such material exchanges between family members take on the characteristics of exchanges between nonkin, it is often a sign that the sense of family has broken down.

Inheritances are forms of gift giving that occur at the time of the giver's death. Like all gift giving, the transfers of money and property involved often convey a great deal of information concerning the relationship between the giver and the recipient. Our laws of inheritance are based on the privileged nature of kin ties, especially those between nuclear family members—father, mother, and children. Rules and patterns of inheritance, like gift giving more generally, can be used to define the boundaries of relationships. When an older person chooses to disinherit a child, the act is tantamount to a declaration that the child is no longer a member of the family. At some basic level, the disinherited person's legitimacy has been revoked.

An example from a case study family probably mirrors many other families' experiences.* Mr. Fairchild disinherited the third of his four daughters for what, in his opinion, were unforgivable transgressions in her young adulthood that hurt him terribly. Mr. Fairchild's daughter had divorced someone whom her father strongly approved of, and for many years father and daughter did not speak. Later, when he was an old man and his daughters well into middle age, Mr. Fairchild's first-born daughter, the executrix of the will, pleaded with him to relent and include the rejected sister in the division of his modest estate. However, his disappointment had been so profound that, although his relationship with this

*The facts in case studies cited throughout this book are true, although the names have been changed to protect the subjects' privacy and identity.

daughter, Candace, had improved, it had changed the demeanor of the kinship tie and formalized an intimate relationship. Perhaps most important, he never reinstated her in his will and he carried his condemnation of her early failures to his grave. His statement was clear; it was also legally irrevocable and eternal.

Examples like this abound even as we enter the dawn of the twenty-first century. For this reason, in this book I investigate the patterns and meaning of household estate wealth that is transferring from the current generation to the next. The issue has taken on significance far beyond what American families and retirees once considered noteworthy, because the country is on the threshold of the largest intergenerational wealth transfer in its history. During our working lives, most of us earn enough money to cover basic living expenses and to care for our dependents. Most middle-class individuals can boast of at least a modest retirement plan and manage to save and invest some money. Others, of course, invest shrewdly and amass large fortunes during their own lifetimes; a very few others win the lottery. For most of us, though, great wealth will forever be a fantasy, and a large fraction of what we acquire through our own efforts is tied up in our home and other personal property (Havens and Schervish, 2003a). On our deaths this property becomes liquid and passes to our heirs.

What follows is an investigation of how different types of families (heirs and testators) with economically and ethnically diverse backgrounds vary in their approaches to handling their assets and the property to be left behind following their death. Both economic and sociocultural variables must be considered if a solid and thoughtful interpretation of the benefactor's allocation of the inheritance is to be achieved. To embark on this journey, I combined quantitative and nonquantitative approaches to the study of gift giving and inheritance from a bigenerational perspective, paying close attention to age-related differences in responses. Many sociologists have moved beyond traditional normative scientific paradigms and embraced multiple research methodologies in their investigations. From my experience, it is clear that both narratives and numbers help to unlock the nuanced meaning of giving acts in mature adulthood. The ultimate goal of the study is to examine the empirical data characterizing the norms and practices of inheritance as one of the material ties between generations and family members. Personal narratives and stories paint a more complete picture of the problems confronting adult children and their parents' generation, greatly enriching the social and moral dimensions underlying patterns in individual behavior in gift giving. These case stories will help to illustrate the intended and unintended social consequences of financial transaction for Baby Boomers and for their parents' generation.

TRENDS IN WEALTH TRANSFERS

Wealth transfers play an important role in our society. To be sure, intergenerational gifts and inheritances are expected to alter the lives of current and future generations in the United States. One has only to look at some statistics on intergenerational wealth transfers to appreciate the magnitude of the effect of this impending event for American families:

- Approximately $25 trillion of wealth will pass from the current generation to the next from the estates of older Americans by the middle of this century (Havens and Schervish, 1999).
- The per capita intergenerational wealth transfer in the United States is about $145,000 (Havens and Schervish, 2003b).
- According to Gale and Scholz (1994), intentional intergenerational transfers and inheritance accounted for about 25 percent of household wealth if transfers such as a child's college tuition or home mortgage are included as a major gift; Kotlikoff and Summers (1981) estimated a larger share, as high as 80 percent.
- Most analysts conclude that about one out of five children will receive bequeathed wealth.

Although typically a death is the impetus that by necessity motivates these transfers, what will be revealed in this study is the transformative effect of many social and noneconomic forces giving rise to new decisions about money matters as the U.S. population ages.

THE AGING AMERICAN FAMILY

Inheritance is increasingly becoming a topic of great interest to many people in the light of the profound demographic changes in aging and family structure witnessed in the past thirty years. Not long ago, older adults had few concerns about how they would handle the transfer of their family financial resources. Intergenerational transfers flowed upward, from adult child to elderly parent, because of the lack of wealth available then to elderly Americans. But the emergence of the *third age*, now commonly defined as older people living well into old age, brings with it an expanded leisure phase of life that has created new imperatives and societal norms for retirement security, as well as new opportunities to pass on assets to the succeeding generations (Laslett, 1991). Population aging has

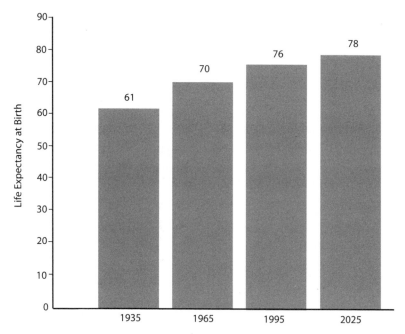

Figure 1.1. Americans Are Living Longer than When Social Security Began
Source: Data from Bipartisan Commission on Entitlement and Tax Reform, 1995.

serious consequences for gift-giving practices between parents and their children and between adult children (Uhlenberg, 1992). This phenomenon is also transforming the character of American social policies, including pension reform and the future of intergenerational transfer programs like Social Security (Hurd and Smith, 2002).

Several factors related to falling death rates, especially among those over 80, will undoubtedly influence family gifts and inheritance practices. To be sure, the biggest demographic change affecting intergenerational relations in the U.S. population is the increased adult life span (Angel and Hogan, 2004). In 1935, an average American lived 61 years (see Figure 1.1). However, because of declining fertility and improvements in medical care, U.S. life expectancy rates in older age groups reached an all-time high in 1995 (Anderton, Barrett, and Bogue, 1997). Today, a 65-year-old woman can expect to live to 84 years and a 65-year-old man to almost 81 years (U.S. Census Bureau, 2006).

That prolonged longevity, married with a large Baby Boom cohort (about 78 million) entering old age, takes on clear relevance for numerous reasons, the most significant of which concerns the economic status of parents and their adult children. Sociologists refer to Americans born roughly during the two decades following World War II as the Baby Boomers. Recent decades have shown a marked increase in the proportion of Baby Boomers whose parents are still alive; as of 1992, slightly more than a third of late middle-age persons had one parent still living (Henretta, Grundy, and Harris, 2001). As a result, as parents are living longer, they are more concerned with having enough assets for their health and retirement than with building a large estate to leave to their children (Myles, 2002). Another looming problem for many American retirees is that the nation's medical care costs continue to soar. In 1960 Americans spent $27 billion, and by 2003 that number had increased to $1.7 trillion. In 2003, the average combined public and private per capita annual expenditure for health care was $5,670, as opposed to $348 just 33 years earlier (1970), when the costs of hospitals, doctors' fees, and inflation were much lower than they are today (Office of the Assistant Secretary for Planning and Evaluation, 2005). Health care will continue to assume a larger fraction of the U.S. gross domestic product; after rising from 5 percent in 1960 to 15 percent in 2003, it is expected to reach 17 percent in 2012.

As Figure 1.2 shows, although Medicare and Medicaid comprise almost one-third of national health care expenditures, in recent years private insurance and out-of-pocket payments have accounted for a larger share of the amount. However, American workers can expect to assume an even greater role in financing their health care. Forty percent of Americans relied on private insurance to cover the costs of medical care in 2005 as opposed to 23 percent in 1960. The second most important source for private health care expenditures is out-of-pocket dollars; 15 percent used personal money to cover his or her medical expenses in 2005. Medicaid is the largest component of state and local governments' expenditures on health care. As a result of rising Medicaid obligations, budgets are being squeezed very tightly, and the cost of higher education is shifting to parents and students (Kane and Orszag, 2003).

An aging society combined with the growing costs of health care will affect inheritance practices, especially as the result of the anticipated increase in the number of years spent with compromised health (Crimmins, Hayward, and Saito, 1996). The rising prevalence of cognitive and physical frailty and disabilities will cause higher costs for medical care and long-term care to manage and treat very old persons with disabling medical conditions (Altman, Reinhardt, and Shields, 1998). More money will be needed to cover medical and long-term care services (Stone, 2000). While there is a high chance that many elderly people will be financially well off and able to cover these health care expenditures, others will incur major debt in retirement (Smith and Kington, 1997). They will not be able

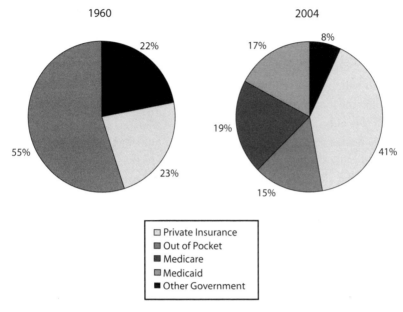

Figure 1.2. Changes in Sources of Financing of Personal Health Care
Source: Data from Assistant Secretary for Planning and Evaluation, 2005.

to afford to pay the insurance premiums, deductibles, and copayments for doctor visits and hospitalization. Even now, medical bills account for half of all personal bankruptcies in the United States (Ostrom, 2004). The economic effects of the consumption of the savings of retired elderly people may be substantial, especially when the financial assets are spent on long-term care. The Health and Retirement Study (HRS), which is conducted by the University of Michigan and supported by the National Institute on Aging, reported that 37 percent to 43 percent of Americans aged 51–61 expect to leave a bequest to their children. It is unknown how a major catastrophic life event such as a disabling medical illness might undermine these good intentions (Mitchell and Moore, 1998; Munnell, Sundén, Soto, and Taylor, 2003).

The *fourth age*, the group defined by some gerontologists as people 85 years and older, is another key family demographic trend affecting gift-giving behavior. Many persons experience physical and cognitive dependency during this period of the life cycle (Wray and Alwin, 2005). As a result, the health consequences associated with this stage of the life course bring an entirely new set of financial issues which elderly persons must confront in deep old age. While many people belonging to this group remain active, a large fraction must face the high costs of disabling illness and long-term care (Hudson, 2005). Extended life expectancies also mean that children tend to be older (and may even be quite elderly themselves) when their parents die (Smith, 2003). The protracted period of aging will no doubt alter the meaning and salience of gifts passed on to adult children, many of whom will themselves be on the cusp of the third age. Longer life spans may mean that the transfer of estates will become a lifelong process rather than something that occurs only on a parent's death.

The effect of aging in the United States on family financial relations is apparent when older parents need long-term care. A recent *New York Times* article highlights the situation of the more than 15 million adult caregivers of aging parents who are increasingly assuming financial responsibility for their parent's home-based long-term care, including both major expenses, like housing, and the often unnoticed out-of-pocket costs such as transportation, clothing, and housekeeping (Gross, 2006). Although the expenses for long-term care may not cause economic hardship for some, many adult children caring for their parents may end up in debt as a result of the financial obligation and the loss of earnings of the caregiver. Many refuse to place a loved one in a nursing home even if they could have afforded to do so.

In addition, dramatic changes in family life in recent decades, including the high divorce rate, influence patterns of intergenerational gifting and inheritance. Research shows that children of divorced parents are much less likely than children of intact families to receive financial and emotional support from their parents (Eggebeen, 1992; Cooney and Uhlenberg, 1992). The period of time away from the father exacerbates the child's situation; the longer the separation, the lower the amount of economic support (Lye, Kleplinger, Hyle, and Nelson, 1995). White, Booth, and Edwards (1992) reach a similar conclusion, finding that remarried divorced parents provide less financial support for their children. What is also becoming more of concern among sociologists and other family scientists is the mountain of evidence indicating that fathers who remarry are predisposed to support their children from the second marriage (McLanahan and Sandefur, 1994) and to give the children from their previous marriage 20 to 25 percent less than they give the children in their new family (White, Booth, and Edwards, 1992).

At the same time, financially well-off grandparents are increasingly a critical source of financial support for their grandchildren (Lewin, 2005). Many of them are also helping their adult children when they struggle to make ends meet. The rising trend in divorce since the 1970s, especially among minority group women, has undermined retirement planning of daughters from the middle class, many of whom did not work and relied solely on their husbands for financial support (Angel, Jiménez, and Angel, 2007).

Perhaps most important, the topic is timely because, for those who can expect to inherit money or property from parents, relatives, or nonkin, a bequest can profoundly alter not only their financial situation but also their self-worth and family relations across the life course. Even relatively modest amounts of money that are above and beyond what one earns can affect one's financial situation measurably. Shapiro (2003) argues that, on balance, gifts of equity (either housing or money) from parents can especially improve the lives and opportunities for generations into the future. This may be one reason that the distribution of a parent's estate can prove conflict-ridden and traumatic for many families, even to the point that it is often fodder for popular drama. One person's good fortune in receiving a tidy bequest is another's loss, and resentments and jealousies even among close family members are not unusual. Occasionally, the division of an estate tears a family apart, and family members can harbor resentments against deceased parents and siblings for years. On the other hand, gift giving in late life can bring great pleasure, allowing reflection by older parents of their generativity and generosity.

For all of the above reasons, inheritance is a particularly salient issue for many Americans approaching retirement and the years beyond.

CHAPTER TWO

The Inheritance Revolution

But the law of inheritance was the last step to equality . . . and *it affects the minds of the heirs and brings their passions into play.*
—*Alexis de Tocqueville*, Democracy in America, 1835

Americans who once thought they would rely mostly on Social Security benefits during retirement are faced with the reality that those funds might not be there. They must now find other sources of money to fill the Social Security gap, should it occur. Inheritances and bequests will play a crucial role in sustaining or creating quality of life for more Americans. This increased importance of inheritance plays out against the changing social landscape of twenty-first-century United States, where life spans are increasing and birth rates are increasing among minorities but decreasing among the majority. The ties that traditionally bound the generations are weakened or nonexistent, affected by blended families and a more mobile society. These social forces need to be explored to define the nature of the family safety net.

Today's beliefs, values, and practices regarding inheritance are nuanced and often complicated. Decisions about what to leave and to whom are colored not only by our personal history but also by our country's laws. How were our current laws and attitudes shaped by our history? How were current inheritance laws conceived, and why were they created? We must go back to our beginnings as an English colony to learn the nature of inheritance laws in the United States.

In traditional societies, inheritance was based on historical practice and common law. One's place in the family and one's claim on one's parents' estate were determined by custom. Rights of inheritance were a reflection of one's position in the social and family hierarchy. In the United States today, the transfer of property is not governed by common practice; one is free to divide one's estate as one wishes. In this context, exchanges are emblematic of one's status in the family rather than vice versa. A historical perspective is especially useful in thinking about the moral values that contribute to our ideals of family gift giving and inheritance practice in the United States.

THE ORIGINS OF OUR INHERITANCE LAWS

In the agrarian American past, the rules surrounding gifts and bequests defined kinship and status and determined the boundaries of family and community. Alexis de Tocqueville understood that U.S. inheritance laws mirrored American attitudes about family independence, obligations, and wealth. As new attitudes evolved, laws and traditions were forged to pass hard-earned wealth, however it was measured, from generation to generation. In 1835, Tocqueville advocated the creation of U.S. estate taxes to level the unfair economic playing field to which he was so accustomed as a French aristocrat (Tocqueville, 1966). In France, as in other European countries, inheritance was simple and effective: the eldest son inherited all real property and his siblings were beholden to him for all their economic prospects. This practice, called primogeniture, arose to avoid the break-up of large estates.

Under the law of primogeniture, land, unlike personal belongings, was not evenly divided among all the children but instead was bequeathed to the oldest son. Therefore, claims on a parent's estate were determined by custom and by one's place in the social and family hierarchy. To be a second or third son, or, worse, a daughter, was to be out of luck.

Primogeniture was incompatible with American political values, according to Tocqueville. In the spirit of family pride, "l'esprit de famille," he believed in and advocated for progressive inheritance tax laws, which could lead to relative financial equality. In his view, equality of inheritance established by law would improve the lives of heirs (including their grand- and great-grandchildren) while maintaining the integrity of the democratic republic espoused by the framers of the U.S. Constitution (Tocqueville, 1990).

EARLY AMERICA

Historians differ on precisely when the "modern American family" emerged. Carl Degler, in his 1980 book *Women and the Family in America from the Revolution to the Present*, traces the development of the modern American family to the years between the American Revolution and about 1830. These years should not be taken precisely; they simply suggest the outer limits of the period of transition from the traditional to the modern family in the United States. The shift was irregular and slow. Generally, American historians, including the late Tamara Hareven, date the emergence of the modern family to the late eighteenth and early nineteenth centuries. By the 1930s, a century later, a form of family had taken shape that was clearly different from that in preindustrial society. Today the American family is built around complementary functions that include an economic unit and emotional roles for mother, father, and children.

In early America, 90 percent of the population was engaged in farming. A husband's ability to command all family assets was the keystone of the family's economic success, and much of that depended on the woman's agreeing to surrender ownership and control of her own inherited assets when she married. Only single women and widows were legally permitted to bequeath property during this period. Their assets were usually small amounts of personal, not real, property. A widow might get the proceeds of the husband's entire estate for a stated period of years if all the children were minors. However, the transfer did not typically occur until the youngest child reached the age of majority. In such cases, even after the estate transferred to the grown children, provision was often made for the widow to receive support.

As mentioned above, primogeniture arose to avoid the breakup of large English estates (Narrett, 1992). The basic nature of real property tenure was transferred to America from England and included all of the following characteristics: ownership of land by purchase was perpetual as long as taxes due were met; land could descend to heirs either by will or by inheritance with or without a will; and land ownership included subsurface as well as surface resources, so mineral rights transferred with the land.

During the colonial period, inheritance practices revealed a significant concern for maintaining an intact family business or farm, much as primogeniture did. Productive assets held by a family were seldom liquidated; they were usually passed on to a surviving son. Other heirs would receive cash or some lesser portion of the tangible property, which included such things as livestock or household goods. Except for the very wealthy, few willed anything much to charity or other relatives. The availability of abundant land influenced inheritance practices, providing more opportunities for the offspring that did not inherit real property.

Sons were still favored over daughters in this system, which reinforced the patriarchal power base and increased wealth differences between men and women (Shammas, Salmon, and Dahlin, 1997). In general, the family estate tended to give real property or "realty" to sons and personal property to daughters. However, by writing a will, a father could make as many stipulations as he wished, such as increasing the daughters' shares to make up for the double share to the eldest son or giving daughters only personal (instead of real) property. A daughter's portion of real property was often for life only and reverted to her brothers when she died; this was intended to prevent her husband (a non-blood relative) from liquidating it and distributing the proceeds outside the family. If upon a husband's death there were no living children, usually the wife received half the estate and the other half went to the husband's relatives.

In the colonial era, a father's control over inheritance kept his grown sons dependent on him for years while they waited to receive the landed property they needed to establish an independent household (Shammas et al., 1997). Likewise, a daughter's dependency on her father for a dowry resulted in little female autonomy. But, rapid population growth and a consequential carving out of plots too small to be farmed viably, weakened paternal control over inheritance. As the colonial period progressed, an increase in opportunities for nonagricultural work allowed men and women to marry earlier than when their sole means of family support derived from agricultural production on inherited real property.

Inheritance probably played a more important role in the economy during the colonial period than at any other time in American history. The economy depended on the family firm or farm almost exclusively, and inheritance determined the distribution of the family's assets among family members. Too wide a distribution of resources and control among successive heirs might jeopardize business operations and would affect the economic welfare of future generations. Keeping a firm or farm intact had its appeal; hence, the need for the customs of primogeniture and, specifically, an "entail" on the conveyed property (to prevent an heir from passing it on) continued.

The foundation of the American inheritance system lies in the European tradition, especially in English laws. English inheritance laws, which governed both the division of property in the absence of a will (intestate inheritance) and the degree of testamentary freedom (disposition of personal property in one's will) possessed by individuals, set the terms for colonial America (Hoffer, 1992). Testamentary rules allotted a double share of the wealth to the oldest son and other male heirs in land and intangibles; daughters typically received a smaller share. In the absence of a will, one-third of the estate or real property (the dower) was given to the widow, and the remaining two-thirds was divided among the children. Thus, as in England, American property owners were overwhelmingly adult white males, which meant that most testators (persons having made a will) were men. Two-thirds of testators who had farms to pass on kept them intact, although doing so demanded much family cooperation. Of the remaining third, most testators divided the productive capital into parcels that were still viable agricultural units.

Not liquidating a landholding meant that the lives of siblings and the widow were tied together for a long time. An eldest son had to buy out any brothers or sisters who chose not to be part of the family business. Widows with only minor children were allowed to manage real property but not sell it, and were required to relinquish the property to the first son who came of age. Older widows had to accept room, living space, and food allotments in a household they had once run, or to live off the income of property they could not alienate (transfer to another person). Daughters received some cash portions of an estate, but there was a price involved there as well: they frequently received less than they would have had there been no will (Shammas et al., 1997).

FORGING A NEW PATH: WOMEN AND INHERITANCE LAWS

In the past, the rules surrounding inter vivos gifts and bequests defined kinship and status within a family (Graeber, 2001). These rules also determined the boundaries of family and community (Becker, 1974). As early as 1750, however, a much higher percentage of the nation's assets were in mercantile and manufacturing enterprises (Cochran, 1985). For this reason, President Jefferson believed that the custom of primogeniture could be abandoned in the new republic and replaced with revised inheritance laws that fostered financial independence, equality in children's inheritance (multigeniture), and widespread participation in government: "The consequences of this enormous inequality producing so much misery to the bulk of mankind, legislators cannot invent too many devices for subdividing property, only taking care to let their subdivisions go hand in hand with the natural affections of the human mind" (Katz, 1977–1978, p. 17). From Jefferson's perspective, land ownership was the bulwark of American democracy and should be passed on from generation to generation in the centuries to come.

For both symbolic and practical reasons, it gave American citizens the economic independence from all political powers. It also aided rapid settlement of estates.

The land ordinances of the mid-1700s laid the foundation of future American capitalism because now land passed into private hands and ended the practice of primogeniture (Salmon, 1986). In the New World, the laws of primogeniture were disallowed in the Old Northwest Ordinance of 1787, as well as in future land policies in the United States, and this favored an increase in the number of American farmers. The U.S. land policy was predominantly focused on small family-farm distribution, as called for by Thomas Jefferson (Libecap and Hansen, 2001). Eventually, the earlier land ordinances were replaced by the Homestead Act of 1862, in which a family could claim between 40 and 160 acres and, after five years, receive title.

With the ending of primogeniture in all states, the distribution of wealth between men and women was equalized, at least from a legal standpoint (Shammas et al., 1997). New forms of financial assets, such as income from rent, made land sales and liquidation easier, probably freeing some siblings from the kind of long-term family obligation that buy-outs had occasioned in the past (Shammas et al., 1997). Most state laws gave all children equal shares rather than giving the eldest a double share. This, of course, could be changed if there was a will. Theoretically, wives still received one-third of the estate, but because they could not own the property outright, it was more often in the form of living space, food, firewood, or a cow for her lifetime, and then only if she remained a widow. The laws about women bequeathing property remained the same. More land was available (e.g., bounty lands) and more families moved westward. At the same time, a higher proportion of families engaged in nonagricultural businesses. Even in 1965, American property owners were still overwhelmingly white males, and the traditional division of property in the absence of a will was one-third to the widow, with the remaining two-thirds divided among the children.

The changing social situation of women gave rise to changes in inheritance practice. Coverture, the legal subordination of a married woman to her husband, prevailed in the United States until the middle of the nineteenth century, when New World economies demanded women's involvement in work. During the industrial revolution, the common law rights, which deprived a wife of her husband's property and any contractual obligations, were eliminated or modified in all states. Most states by statute provided the surviving spouse with a right to one-third or one-half of the decedent's estate, without regard to sex. Legislative acts governing married women's property rights, passed in England in 1870 and at various times in the United States, gave women control over their own property (Salmon, 1986). The first states to enact legislation overriding the disabilities associated with coverture did so in 1839. Such legislation established the rights of women to enjoy the profits of their labor, to control real and personal property, to be parties to lawsuits and contracts, and to execute wills on their own behalf. Most property rights for women emerged in piecemeal fashion over the course of decades. New states were coming into the union, and many of them enacted community property laws so that both spouses shared equally in the income earned and property acquired during the marriage. Among the first "community property states" were Arizona, California, Idaho, Louisiana, Nevada, New Mexico, Texas, and Washington. In time, many states enacted similar laws, and most states passed women's property acts.

Because judges frequently interpreted the statutes narrowly, women had to agitate for more expansive and detailed legislation, such as specification of the right of a married woman to maintain ownership and control over real and personal property she had inherited or had been given, and the right to bequeath or give such property to whom she chose. Although eventually daughters received equal shares with sons, again, that could be changed by a will. Most states required parents to put their intentions in writing in a will if they planned to disinherit a son or daughter. If a parent died intestate (without a will), all children inherited equally.

Interestingly, there were cultural differences in women's right to wealth between the Native Americans and the rest of the American population. In both Iroquois and Algonkian societies, women held powers and rights not granted in English society, including the right to inherit property.

INHERITANCE IN MODERN AMERICA

As the nation's customs, population, and technology evolved, patterns of inheritance changed (Shammas et al., 1997). By the time of the industrial revolution, the changing nature of property from traditional to contemporary societies had transformed American families. The U.S. Constitution outlawed primogeniture and entail (the practice of leaving everything to the eldest son) in 1789, thus opening up new ways to transfer wealth.

Even today, the transfer of property is not governed by common practice but is determined by testamentary freedom—people are free to divide their estates as they wish. In this situation, exchanges define one's position in the family rather than the other way around. Wealth transmission among middle-class families tends to center on cash assets transferred during a parent's life course (inter vivos gifts, ones between living people) and far less on transfers of the "family farm or family firm" by inheritance (Langbein, 1988, p. 723). Today, we view property and money as material goods that can be bought, sold, or given away with impunity (Hashimoto, 1996). For American billionaires, such as Ted Turner, Warren Buffett, and Bill Gates, new fortunes have resulted in a new "ethos of inheritance," emblematic of what it takes to remain competitive in a global economy. The advanced industrialized nations flourished after World War II, and decisions about inheritance of the resulting massive accumulation of wealth shifted from the notion of patrimony to an increase in the investments in human capital associated with modern economies. The desire and need to obtain a high-quality education for children, especially in institutions of higher learning, has replaced transfer of family possessions (assets, such as a home, business, stocks and bonds) after a parent's death as the pathway by which Americans convey their wealth to their children.

Hall and Marcus (1998), on the other hand, note that what marks the watershed of the inheritance revolution is actually the lack of "inheritance ethos" exhibited by the wealthiest Americans, who tend to think of the short-term rather than long-term implications of their spending during their life time. Widespread credit card debt, ownership of two homes, and an inculcated taste for consumption of amenities, are mortgaging not only the future of families in the United States but also social institutions and the community at large. The prevailing attitudes toward conventional modes of inheritance to some extent, then, as Miller and McNamee (1998) observe, can undermine the basic foundation of society and as a result the next generation's lives by destroying physical capital and, ultimately, slowing the pace of long-term economic growth.

The exchange of material goods and money is not so simple. While it is true that most middle-class parents embody the emotional commitment to help their children, the notion of the "new ethos" may actually apply to contemporary American parents of even modest means. Clearly, in the future, consumption behavior in middle age will take on new meaning, as more wealth transmission occurs during one's lifetime (Miller and McNamee, 1998). Parents today are so interested in conspicuous achievement, spending hundreds of thousands of dollars on their children's higher education because they associate price with quality, that they are willing to forgo providing an inheritance for their children (Glater and Finder, 2006). Fortunately, almost three-quarters of parents with children at four-year colleges pay less than full fare for the college of their choice because of heavily discounted prices offset by the colleges' private endowments. And so, while the cost of tuition, board, and fees is rising faster than inflation, many low-income and middle-class families are able to afford the cost of elite colleges because of student aid received from the college. They also take advantage of federal or state student loan programs.

Money and wealth in all their forms are complex symbols, and their exchange is profoundly moral in the sense that it defines the relationship between the giver and the recipient. In a very real sense, our emotional ties are intimately linked to material exchanges. The parent-child bond is strong, and the nature of exchanges between these two generations defines our very social structure. Again, unlike in earlier times, when family wealth depended on inheritance of land by children, the extended life span provides opportunities to transfer assets before parents' deaths to those entitled to succeed.

Social changes to women's inheritance right increased opportunities for securing children's economic well-being. The new laws, aimed at improving women's social status and life chances, presented no gender boundaries. Profound demographic and historical change has affected family life; in the last few decades, major social policy has opened up new roles for women. For example, Title IX of the Educational Equity Act required gender equality in educational opportunities, making it possible for more women to attend college and university. These social and policy changes affected the ways in which parents viewed their legacy and prompted them to view it on a shorter time horizon. Family wealth could now be spent on helping daughters improve their life chances by acquiring human capital in young adulthood, through education and training. And it worked. In 1972, the year Title IX was signed, women earned just 7 percent of all law degrees; in 1977, women earned only 9 percent of all medical degrees. By 1997, however, they received 44 percent of law degrees and 42 percent of medical degrees. In 1977, only a quarter of all Ph.D. degrees went to women. Twenty years later, women earned 41 percent of all Ph.D.s. It is clear from these data that women do not need to limit their aspirations to the role of housewife but can compete effectively with their male counterparts in the labor force (Padavic and Reskin, 2002).

Inheritance and intergenerational obligations, then, go far beyond the transfer of material possessions. It is important, therefore, to uncover the key factors governing such exchanges: who gives to whom, when, and why, and the impact such gifts have on recipients' life chances and education and on family relations. The implications that income flows have on the inner workings of family life, on the establishment of meaningful personal legacies, and on meeting societal needs are also useful.

FAMILY AND INHERITANCE CHANGES

What is the contemporary view and role of inheritance in the United States? Although the broad issue of inheritance has intrigued many historians, economists, sociologists, lawyers, and other researchers, few empirical data exist today to tell us much about how changes in the transmission of wealth can transform family lives. Marvin Sussman, a well-known sociologist, argues (1970) that much of the work on income transfers examines systems of maintenance and care for sustaining the economic well-being of the family at an aggregate level. At the societal level, he contends, "financial support of social security welfare and education by persons in their middle years may be interpreted as a legacy for the younger and older generations" (p. 3). At the same time, leaving a personal legacy to a child may be observed at the individual level. From this perspective, parents define the meaning of kin interactions and relationships through transfers of their property to another family member in a will (bequest).

The corporate structure of modern economic systems reduces the necessity for an orderly intergenerational transfer of equity within family and kinship lines to enhance the continuity of the economic system, a prerequisite in the preindustrial period. The preponderance of evidence suggests that economic growth weakens the bond among extended families owing to the ascendancy of the nuclear family (Becker, 1974). And because people no longer live in extended households of multiple generations of adults, property flows from parents to children as opposed to going from children to parents (Altonji, Hayashi, and Kotlikoff, 1997; Cox, 1987).

For more than thirty years, scholars such as Becker (1974) and Barro (1974) have argued that the demographic transition from high birth and death rates to low fertility and mortality increases economic development and creates a crowding-out effect, in which private old-age supports are replaced by public transfers. In some respects, this is true. To be sure, the considerable influences of government-sponsored programs such as Social Security, disability insurance, and health care entitlements have reduced the importance of inheritance to the economic maintenance of the family in modern times (Mitchell and Moore, 1998). However, the transfer of property in modern industrial nations is still a vital function as evidenced in the new family economy (Pestieau, 2003). The family as the social safety net is still a major source of support for many Americans.

One of its manifestations is a change in the intergenerational transfer of resources. In the United States, inheritances make up the majority of personal wealth (Havens and Schervish, 2002). The booming stock and real estate markets of the 1990s created wealth at an extraordinary rate. That trend is adding trillions of dollars to the vast amount of wealth that will be passed on to a new generation of heirs during the next twenty years. The majority of estates are still distributed through inheritance, resulting in an increase in the number of families affected by the estate tax, and this could create a groundswell of popular support for repealing, or at least easing, the estate tax.

A speculative study in 1999 by the Social Welfare Research Institute at Boston College concludes that, from 1998 through 2018, the parents of Baby Boomers and some aging Boomers themselves will leave estates worth a mind-boggling $12 trillion to $18 trillion, creating the largest generational transfer of wealth in history. According to the study, that enormous wealth transfer will include as many as 2.8 million estates worth $1 million or more (Havens and Schervish, 1999).

But, property transfers will not benefit everyone equally. African Americans and Latinos were largely excluded from participation in the developing economy and their adaptations to exclusion have produced another source of family variation. Ethnic diversity has become more pronounced as many immigrants from non-European nations enter the United States. From 1980 to 1990, the total Hispanic population of the United States increased by 53.0 percent, and the black population increased by 13.2 percent (as compared to increases of 6.0 percent for whites). These high rates of growth for that decade (exceeded only by the Asian-American population, 99 percent) raised the percentage of the total non-white U.S. population to 19.7 percent (Anderton, Barrett, and Bogue, 1997).

It is important to recognize here that being black, Hispanic, or immigrating as an adult in late life adversely influences the accumulation of assets, and that ultimately a lack of social capital undermines one's access to resources in retirement (Angel and Angel, 2006; Crystal and Shea, 2003). These fundamental levels of income inequality plague minorities and women, particularly in terms of inheritance, savings accounts, stocks, bonds, home equity, and other investments (Angel and Angel, 1997; Holden and Smock, 1991; Wolff, 2003).

Once again, with the increasing number of Americans, especially women, entering the third age of life, it is important to understand the retirement behavior of ethnically diverse groups. Clearly, an assessment of the economic situation of vulnerable and disadvantaged populations requires our attention.

DECISIONS ABOUT INHERITANCE

Although we tend to think of wills as a common financial planning tool with which to pass on wealth, research indicates that wills were rare before the twentieth century (Curran, 1989). Testation, the act of writing a will, evolved in the administration of estates under statutory authority as surviving spouses have assumed the principal roles of both executor and beneficiary in most contemporary wills (Dukeminier and Johanson, 2000). A will is created so that the testator, the person making the will, may bequeath assets to specific persons. Before the twentieth century, when most people did not create wills, probate courts were created in an attempt to locate all family survivors so that the state (or colony) could determine the legal distribution of the deceased's estate. The county court was responsible for the distribution of property after the death of its owner, whether or not there was a will.

Today, while many Americans do die intestate, a national survey conducted in 1994 found that among elderly people, 70 percent of persons age 70–85 reported having wills (O'Connor, 1996). However, even many wealthy, well-educated persons do not adequately prepare a will. A few years ago, former U.S. Supreme Court Justice Warren Burger died without writing a formal will. He did not consult a fellow attorney who specialized in wills. He failed to provide for estate taxes and to include a grant of powers to his executor; his self-written 176-word will cost his heirs because he failed to give any power to his executors (Carelli, 1995). These apparent oversights cost the estate thousands of dollars. Naturally, one would have thought that such a distinguished jurist and brilliant legal authority would be the last person to make such an unfortunate oversight. Billionaire Howard Hughes wrote many wills, but at the time of his death, none of them indicated exactly who should inherit his wealth. In each of these two cases, lack of an adequate will caused significant expense and inconvenience to their respective families. The reluctance to prepare a will may be a result of the unique situation of the very wealthy; while they are likely to be concerned with the long-term maintenance of family assets, they generally have little hesitation about liquidating such assets. Now, offspring are older and better educated, and so are better established in their chosen careers when their parents die (Angel and Hogan, 2004).

Most people without wills indicate that they simply haven't gotten around to the task; it's not something that many individuals happily put on the top of their "to do" lists. But underlying that procrastination is the belief that, upon one's unexpected death, without a valid will, things will somehow work out—one's assets will go to the people whom one intends to receive them or to those who want to receive them.

Often, parents make wrong assumptions about estate planning, and one such assumption is goodwill among family members. Many factors, including the rising number of step-parent families, strong attitudes of Depression-era parents about holding onto their inheritance, and debt-ridden Baby Boomers, have strained family relations (Fish and Kotzer, 2002). Many internecine problems arise when wealth passes from generation to generation. To be sure, family harmony is the most commonly overlooked aspect of inheritance planning (Greene, 2002).

In summary, the transition from family to corporate capitalism had several origins, including the decline in birth rate, the increased role of the state, and the emergence of intangible (particularly financial) forms of wealth. These changes redefined trends in American family norms and the law. First, a smaller percentage of the U.S. population earns its living from farming. Second, upon death, assets are usually liquidated and the proceeds divided equally among children and other descendants. Third, under current law, trusts and other schemes may be established to avoid taxes imposed on inheritance, gifts, and generation-skipping wealth transfers for upper-income families (Kopczuk and Slemrod, 2003). Finally, and most significantly, statutes have been enacted that equalize the position of widows and widowers and improve the position of both at the expense of children. Today, in most states, the traditional life estate unconditionally passes to the widow in the event her husband dies intestate. In 1945, the federal Administration of Estates Act (Section 45) abolished the common law dower, a fixed portion of a deceased husband's estate allotted by law to his widow for her lifetime. Abolishing the requirement of a husband's permission before a wife could sell her property was important because women, especially those from middle-class families, relied primarily on their husbands for economic support.

The position of women as inheriting daughters, surviving spouses, or as testators has improved. Women have acquired the same property rights as men, widows are in the same position as widowers, and the tendency to favor sons over daughters has diminished. Nonetheless, affluent men are less generous to their female heirs than are male testators of average wealth (Shammas et al., 1997).

The understanding that property from the older generation would be transferred to children with an assumption that they would support their parents in old age is much less prevalent than it once was. Economic affluence and financial independence of children from their parents at an earlier age, coupled with societal mechanisms for economic transfers, have shifted the primary motivators for parental care to the emotional sphere—for affection, gratitude, guilt, or desire for approval. The quality of relationships between generations has undergone dramatic changes, and current family roles may have created greater strain on family care systems for elderly people (Treas, 1977).

What follows is an investigation of how different types of family members (heirs and testators) with economically and ethnically diverse backgrounds vary in their approaches to handling their assets and the property to be left behind following their death. In many cases, the cultural significance of inheritance and inter-generational resource flows may become less obvious, although this issue remains to be seen. I compare the current institutional arrangements of U.S. pension programs with those of other industrialized nations, such as Sweden, France, and Italy, which are also undergoing dramatic demographic change in caring for their elderly citizens. The comparison of the old-age welfare states in Europe and the United States helps illuminate the goal of policies designed to influence individual-level accumulation of wealth.

CHAPTER THREE

The Political Realities of Retirement Security

In our every deliberation, we must consider the impact of our decisions on the next seven generations.

—*The Great Law of the Iroquois Confederacy*

As the elderly population increases, social and political pressures are being felt at every level of society, from the kitchen table to the corporate board room. As one generation is poised to collect Social Security, another is being told there won't be enough money to fund their retirement. Consequently, personal savings and inheritances will play an even more vital role in sustaining future generations of Americans. As this chapter illustrates, this situation is not isolated to the United States.

This chapter examines the political factors influencing a family's access to different types of wealth, either private or public, and how they may directly influence one's well-being and ultimately affect family relationships. The analysis focuses specifically on political context, including actors inside and outside of government.

In framing the basic issue of what happens in a society, when the population has greater longevity and a generous social welfare system, one can turn to an international perspective to learn how other nations cope. My argument rests on the assumption that, while most developed nations provide their retired citizens with a package of substantial health and welfare benefits, regardless of income, it may be difficult to do so in the future under the current demographic regime. Increasingly, the capacity of the state to provide some adequate level of financial support to all older adults is problematic because the elderly population itself continues to age and their needs far outweigh what government can fund. Consequently, the family may function as a social safety net. On the other hand, elderly parents may not be able meet the expectations of creating a secure retirement for themselves or for their adult children.

WHO IS GOING TO CARE FOR US?

Understanding the role of the public sector is important because the welfare state is a central component of old-age security. Many nations face major challenges in financing the retirement and health care needs of the Baby Boom Generation. Although addressing such problems will be painful in the short term, the crisis is historically unique and limited. As the Baby Boomers pass from the scene so will the crisis. A far more serious potential problem arises from the ethnic and racial overlay to the age grading of our society. Although the population over the age of 65 is growing more racially and ethnically diverse, the fact that minority populations will remain young means that well into the twenty-first century the racial and ethnic composition of different age strata will vary dramatically. In the future, the younger-age strata will be disproportionately minority and the older strata disproportionately non-minority with non-Hispanic whites remaining in the majority even by the year 2050 (U.S. Census Bureau, 2003).

In essence, the public sector may promote or hinder the old-age welfare state. Yet, for many Americans approaching retirement, the family is still the safety net (Soldo and Freedman, 1994). This is an important distinction to draw because access to private pensions, savings, housing assets, and Social Security affects the relationships between birth cohorts, between the state and the family, and between older parents and adult children. In light of the challenges posed by population aging, how, then, do the state, family, and individuals support people during risky times? Why is the United States so different in its approach to ensuring the welfare of its elders?

THE POLITICAL ECONOMY OF GIVING AND RECEIVING

The U.S. government differs from those of other developed countries in terms of the services it provides to the public, including health services and other forms of financial support. Many problems that are not found in other developed coun-

TABLE 3.1
Retirement Income Security Systems

Country	Poverty Rate as Percentage of GDP (1992)	Guaranteed Minimum as Percentage of Median National Income (1992)	Social Retirement Pensions as Percentage of GDP (1995)	(2030)
United States	13.4	22.7	34	4.1
Germany	4.5	8.1	52	11.1
United Kingdom	10.9	30.5	43	4.5
Canada	1.5	7.1	56	5.2
Australia	7.1	28.6	51	2.6
Netherlands	3.0	4.4	66	6.0
Sweden	1.5	6.4	63	11.8

Source: Adapted from Smeeding and Smith, 1998.

tries, such as infant mortality, are high in the United States. After World War II, welfare states appeared in Western Europe, for instance, in Sweden and the United Kingdom. These nations provide a constellation of services related to family well-being ranging from housing to nutrition. This constellation provides a bulwark of social and health services.

Unlike these Western European nations, the United States does not provide universal entitlement programs offering family allowances, child allowances, housing allowances, child support, early childhood care, food stamps, health services, and parental leave. The Family and Medical Leave Act of 1993 includes the right to leave without pay, which differs significantly from the paid leave offered to Western Europeans (U.S. Department of Labor, 2000). Some programs in these areas, including housing allowances and food stamps, do exist, but they are means tested. Why is the United States so different from Western European nations?

Table 3.1 compares retirement security systems in seven developed nations. It also shows that income inequality will probably increase in the years to come. As the Baby Boom Generation arrives at retirement age, benefit cuts that will almost inevitably be necessary will have their most serious impact on African Americans and Latinos, and especially African American and Latino women, because so many depend on Social Security alone for their economic security (Herd, 2006). In the future, the minority elderly will find themselves particularly dependent on Medicaid.

The twentieth century brought a new level of income security for the aged, a way of life emblematic of the middle class. But families and individuals differ in many important respects that will affect their economic, housing, and medical care needs in old age. When and how each group arrived in the United States—for work, family reunification, or political reasons—and the degree of their economic and cultural assimilation or integration will determine their health, their wealth, their social support, and the social and health services they are likely to need and use (Borjas, 1994; Palloni, Soldo, and Wong, 2002). Some groups, especially immigrant adults, face serious barriers to health care, especially preventive care, because they lack a usual source of care or health insurance (Wallace and Gutierrez, 2005). While Medicare has eliminated many disparities among elderly Americans, differences in access to high-quality health care and long-term care services persist. Demographic processes and changes in the cultural composition of each age stratum have profound implications for all age groups and for the demands that elderly people will place on our health care system and on other formal and informal sources of support (Estes and Associates, 2001).

THE LEGACY OF THE MODERN WELFARE STATE

Providing pensions and health coverage for elderly people is an important public policy priority in many nations. Worldwide, the aged receive support from three sources: (1) state pension, (2) employer pension, and (3) private savings. Looming costs from the Baby Boom Generation in the United States and elsewhere, as well as general aging of the population, have put a major focus on adapting these programs in order to contain costs. Danish political sociologist Gøsta Esping-Andersen has a typology of social welfare in postindustrial societies that best summarizes these approaches. Table 3.2 draws from his work (1990, 1996, 1999) to elucidate how social welfare policy and the "welfare state" have evolved. The table presents a typology of welfare states classified in terms of their regime characteristics.

Esping-Andersen argues that life involves risks, some of which, like cancer, heart disease, unemployment, poverty, disability, and premature death, can be unpredictable and do not affect everyone. Other risks, such as old age, chronic illness, and functional decline, are much more predictable and affect everyone to some degree. The question, therefore, is Who is responsible for dealing with these risks? There are three possible answers, and nations differ in the extent to which they rely on each:

- the family and the individual;
- the market; or
- the state, by which we mean a collective body of government.

The family's traditional responsibilities involve: The care of children and elderly people. Health care also belongs to the family sphere, as well as household produc-

TABLE 3.2
Academic Typology of Modern Welfare States

"Liberal" Minimal Welfare Model
- Minimize the state's role
- Seek to individualize risks and promote market solutions
- Do not favor citizen entitlements
- Social welfare programs are focused on "bad risks"
- A fairly narrow definition of who is eligible
- Means testing is common
- Emerge where Christian Democratic or Socialist movements are weak
- *Examples:* United States, Australia, New Zealand, Canada

Social Democratic (Scandinavian) Welfare States
- Characterized by universalism
- Comprehensive risk coverage
- Generous benefit levels and income maintenance
- Egalitarianism (including of gender)
- Fusion of welfare and work; full employment guarantee
- Minimize the family (state assumes responsibility for social services)
- Emerge from a strong Social Democratic tradition
- Growing tax burden, but social policies favor the young over the old
- *Examples:* Denmark, Norway, Sweden

Conservative Welfare States (Social Insurance Model)
- Display status segmentation and corporatism (distinct social classes)
- Defend the family and traditional social distinctions
- Male breadwinner model; women discouraged from working
- Little concern with egalitarianism
- Emerge in countries with strong Christian Democratic or conservative coalitions (sometimes with a fascist interregnum)
- Evolved from a tradition of monarchical "etatism" or state socialism
- *Examples:* Germany, Austria, France, Italy

Source: Adapted from Esping-Andersen, 1990.

tion of goods and services like clothes manufacture, food production and preparation, laundry, haircuts, etc. These were all consumed in the family household.

In terms of the market for social services, what was at one time dealt with by the extended family is now relegated to the market. Examples of these goods and services include private or employer-based life and health insurance. In a rapidly aging population, the modern health care system consists of an acute-chronic care continuum across the life course. It includes day care, home health care, assisted living facilities, and nursing home care. The purchase of services by working parents may include child care, domestic services, and personal services like a concierge.

But there are serious gaps in this system. For example, the unemployed, the poor, the mentally ill, the uneducated, the frail old, single mothers, the disabled, and the like are uninsurable, and most cannot purchase these services. In these situations, the state is the insurer of last resort (Institute of Medicine, 2004) Increasingly, and to varying degrees, the state assumes the role of the family in dealing with those risks that the market cannot absorb (Soldo and Freedman, 1994).

As Table 3.2 shows, nations differ in the degree to which their welfare policies emphasize the family, the market, or the state. The Nordic countries are heavily state-based and deemphasize the family's responsibility while guaranteeing the costs of an extensive social service array tailored to individual and parental expectations of needs and tastes. Although social and health care entitlements in the Scandinavian welfare states are equalized across income groups, they are nevertheless adjusted for the discriminating preferences of middle- and upper-income classes and strive for high-quality service delivery. The Mediterranean nations and Japan focus on the family. "Liberal" welfare state regimes, such as the United States, prefer market solutions (Esping-Andersen, 1990). Within the United States, labor-based political parties tend to favor state guaranteed entitlements, while conservative parties prefer to rely on the market. Christian Democratic parties and the religious right wish to deemphasize both the market and the state and reinforce the family. For all three welfare systems, a rapidly growing older population combined with a shrinking labor force will put a strain on public resources.

Unlike the social democratic welfare regime, the problem of inequality plagues the "liberal" welfare states, which primarily provide public assistance cash and medical benefits based on a means test, which is aimed at poor or near-poor family households. As a result, health care services under Medicaid benefits for poor families and infirm older adult recipients are often impoverished and highly stigmatized. However, the other tier of the minimal welfare regime consists of a social insurance system that provides health care and pension benefits based on an age test. In the latter system, the state offers a minimum guaranteed retirement income and medical benefits (hospitalization and physician services) for Social Security–covered workers while affluent middle-class Americans enjoy what the market can provide in terms of higher-quality social and health care services.

THE DILEMMA

There is a growing disjuncture between existing institutional arrangements and emerging population risk profiles. Most welfare regimes were, until recently, based on a male-breadwinner model. The great rural-to-urban migration of the nineteenth and twentieth centuries consisted of families in which the wife did not enter the labor force full-time. Today, most women have entered the workforce.

How do welfare states, then, respond to the new postindustrial reality? Below, I describe key differences between nations, based on important concepts such as entitlement and means-tested programs, and taxation policies (e.g., visible versus invisible taxes).

There are many cultural values that explain the U.S. position, including an emphasis on personal responsibility, a weakened level of trust in government, and a weakened labor movement in the country (Esping-Andersen, 2002). The programs operated by the United States for children and families include, but are not limited to, Temporary Aid to Needy Families (TANF), Medicaid (health care for low-income families and low-income elderly people), Women Infants and Children (WIC), Maternal Child Health Block Grants, Food Stamps, housing assistance, and the National School Lunch Program (Angel and Angel, 1993). In contrast to the programs offered for children and families, there are three large initiatives related to older people: Social Security, Medicare, and Supplemental Security Income (SSI), a cash assistance program serving old people, blind people, and people with disabilities who have very low income (Crystal and Shea, 2003). The programs established for families and children differ from the policies crafted for elderly people in part because poverty is stigmatized in this country (Angel and Angel, 1993). The middle class views entitlements that benefit elderly people as a reward for citizenship and for having contributed to society (Estes, 1979), but entitlements that help low-income families with children are not viewed with the same generosity. In the end, there is an idea that some low-income individuals are worthy or deserving of assistance but others are not. Because U.S. citizens fear a large state, the notion of an expanded welfare state is resisted highly.

EMPLOYER PENSION VERSUS PERSONAL SAVINGS

Even when workers save for retirement through employer pension funds, the end result may be bitter. When President Gerald Ford signed the Employee Retirement Income Security Act thirty years ago, it was supposed to keep pension fund insolvencies from happening. The law, known as ERISA of 1974, requires companies that offer pensions to set aside money to secure the benefits. Companies are not supposed to guess: they must follow a detailed set of rules in calculating contributions (Langbein and Wolk, 2004). The U.S. Department of Labor shows that many corporations are defaulting on their pension plans, despite the regulations protecting employees under the federal law (Walsh, 2005).

Added to the fragility of employer-sponsored pension programs is the issue of whether individuals are disciplined enough or can afford to put aside money for retirement. Why is it that some households save so little while others of the same social class appear to accumulate so much wealth, making it possible to pass on assets to their children and to others? Do individuals save primarily to bequeath to their heirs, to reconcile differences in the timing of income and consumption over the life cycle, or to insure against future uncertainty regarding income, employment, or health? In the absence of state support, will elderly parents alter their personal savings behavior and/or consumption patterns before and during retirement years, including what they transfer to their children?

For most older individuals, a middle-class existence depends on having a private pension (Wise, 1996). A private pension represents an important part of a package that includes Social Security benefits and income from assets (Crystal and Shea, 2003). Without income from a private pension, an older individual's economic security remains precarious, because the maximum monthly Social Security benefit for an individual in 2003 was $1,741 (Social Security Administration, 2006) and most individuals receive much less. In November 2004 the average payment was only $929.40 (Social Security Administration, 2006). According to data from the Survey of Consumer Finances, while 53.7 percent of non-Hispanic white households owned retirement accounts in 1998, only 32.1 percent of nonwhite households were vested in such plans (Aizcorbe, Kennickell, and Moore, 2003). This low rate of pension plan participation by minority households means that the economic security of a large proportion of older minority Americans rests on a single pillar and they face a high risk of an inadequate retirement income (Honig, 2000).

The literature on accumulation of wealth explores several concepts. The life-cycle model indicates that individuals save for later life when they have extra funds. This model, while well backed in the literature, had empirical problems, and so several models were created to account for uncertainty and how people manage and save their funds in relation to the future. Several models focus on bequests and predict that bequests will decrease over time. Rationality is also a focus in the literature, and it provides a framework to explain savings. There are several recurring research questions related to this issue, including:

- Do elderly people save or not?
- What is the motivation for bequests?
- How do social insurance programs change household savings and wealth?
- What is the relationship between private pensions and wealth?
- When does consumption occur in relation to retirement?
- How do capital gains affect savings?
- How do health care prices relate to the accumulation of wealth?

- How does tax policy affect savings?
- Do elderly people use wealth from housing?
- What is the relationship between wealth and labor decisions?
- How do demographics affect the stock market?

Previously, the consumption data required to do thorough analysis of retirement wealth was not available, because collection of information is time-consuming and the results are often biased to underreport consumptive behaviors. Many countries have not even collected these data, because they consider the information to be too private to ask citizens. The availability of new paneled data in the United States, Japan, and Europe make the examination of these issues possible, though there remains a need for better data.

Basic differences exist in how countries finance their retirement plans; differing foci are public, private, and personal funds. The type of public policy option pursued by a government affects private savings. For example, if a public program is expansive, people will save less. For the many nations with baby boom crises, pay-as-you-go plans will face inevitable crunches. Poverty for elderly people is high in the United States and other places where the safety net is minimal. The recommendations from this chapter include gathering better micro-level data to illustrate the connection among income, wealth, retirement incentives, health, and wealth transfers, developing new ways to collect these data, and using the data to determine the effects of public policies on wealth and savings.

CROSS-NATIONAL RESEARCH

I next turn to the presentation of empirical evidence on ways in which public transfer programs and policies can influence personal savings and other family behaviors. Support of these assertions comes from the Organization for Economic Co-operation and Development (OECD) and the Luxembourg Income Study. These data allow a cross-national comparison of the current institutional arrangements of U.S. pension programs with those of other industrialized nations, for example Sweden, France, and Italy, who are also undergoing dramatic demographic changes in caring for their elderly citizens.

The comparison of the old-age welfare systems in Europe and the United States helps to illuminate the goal of public policies designed to influence individual-level wealth accumulation. For example, although the state is often viewed as the safety net for older people in developed countries, as Chapter 2 showed, increasingly many middle-class divorcees are turning to family for support, because they are entering their retirement years without any private wealth or substantial assets (Angel, Jiménez, and Angel, 2007).

As mentioned, worldwide, the aged receive support from the state, the market, and the family. Family support is the focus of the analysis in this study. Adults often provide their parents with the support they provide to their children financially, in terms of time, and in terms of care. The level of support provided within the family varies from country to country; in Asia, this support is high while in Scandinavia, this support is low. The United States falls between these extremes. Demographic crises in many nations have occurred because the number of aged individuals is increasing and there are fewer individuals able to support them financially.

State-provided and family-provided sources of assistance are related, but it is often hard to predict how changes in one level of care will affect the other. Several significant policy questions related to this relationship warrant further review. First, do state programs trade off with family contributions? Second, how do bequests influence transfers of wealth from elderly people to their children? Third, do aged persons enjoy more privacy and independence with increased wealth? Fourth, what are the costs of caregiving to the individual and the state? Fifth, how can policy initiatives spur savings in middle or late life? Finally, how do social policies designed to effect opportunities in early life structure one's life choices and decisions in late life? The policy options that potentially affect personal wealth include encouraging private savings, encouraging later retirement, and encouraging help from relatives.

In the attempt to understand wealth accumulation, several models have been formulated. Samuelson developed a model in 1958 called the overlapping generations model, in which the young work and the older populations retire (Samuelson, 1958). Arthur and McNicoll (1978) created a better version of this model, using age and time as continuous variables and examining the connection between population growth and per capita consumption over a lifetime. Caldwell (1976) examined wealth flows and development and found that in countries with high fertility, the transfers were more from the young to the old; low-fertility countries had more transfer from old to young. This research has identified the primary differences in wealth patterns in the United States and in developing nations. First, in developed countries, individuals consume more than they produce. Second, in developed countries, population growth and mortality are low, so the group of dependent young people is smaller than in developing countries.

To understand wealth transfers between generations, it is important to map the kin network. This process will yield a better understanding of the arrangements of individual families and define the elderly individual and his or her relatives. Surveys to yield this information can take two forms, individual-centered surveys and exchange-centered models. To improve the kin-mapping process, analysts map kin networks, identify individuals who provide different levels of support, and distinguish between what services are provided to each spouse. If supports involving many people distinguish between who gets what, they examine lifetime transfers of wealth instead of current transfers, focus on transfers of financial resources and time within families, and examine other forms of assistance, like emotional assistance, that are not easily quantified.

Because of the expected rise in health care costs over the next couple of years (national health care spending is estimated to double between 2002 and 2012, from $1.5 trillion to $3.1 trillion), there has been an increased focus on mapping both the family structure and behavioral patterns (Heffler et al., 2003). Over the decade beginning in 2002, that will equal $5,427 per capita, or 14.8 percent of a GDP of about $10.5 trillion, compared with $9,972 per capita, or 17.7 percent of a projected GDP in 2012 of about $17.4 trillion. These models can focus on characteristics of household heads, household structure and living arrangements, and kin networks, marital status transitions, and other variables often derived from in-depth survey data.

With regard to kinship network analysis, there are two streams in the literature. First, there is a macro level of analysis that focuses on intergenerational models of demographic and economic processes. Public transfers from younger taxpayers to retirees will be offset by private transfers from parents to their children, so that net savings are unchanged. Microanalysis, while richer, is often not possible, due to a lack of data concerning nations other than the United States, especially other developing countries. Measures of the portion of the total national income that goes to various segments of the population (e.g., quintiles) show that U.S. wage distribution was the most unequal when compared with other advanced capitalist countries. In the United States in 2005, the top 20 percent of households earned 50 percent of the pretax income while the bottom 40 percent earned only 12 percent of income. Perhaps more important, the top 5 percent owned more than half of all wealth in the United States (DeNavas-Walt, Proctor, and Lee, 2006). In 1998, Americans in the top 20 percent owned about 80 percent of all wealth. According to Wolff (2003), overall wealth inequality has grown in the past thirty years and today the bottom 20 percent of family households have either no assets or savings, and massive credit card or medical care debt that exceeds their liquid assets. Some of the main causes of the greater gap between poor and wealthy citizens in the United States and other industrialized nations are declining wages among the working poor, less disposable income among the poor, and the large number of female-headed families who comprise roughly two-fifths of the bottom quintile.

As a consequence, the U.S. government does less in terms of tax and transfer policy to cushion the disparities (Smeeding, Rainwater, and Higgins, 1990). What this evidence portends, then, is a growing level of income inequality of the United States during retirement compared to industrial nations that have a much higher percentage, about 80 percent, of disposable income replaced during retirement (Organization for Economic Co-operation and Development, 1998).

In summary, nations differ on the political structure and policy options that govern the transfer of wealth. It is clear that public policies and socioeconomic conditions affect intergenerational financial relationships, and the opportunities to pass on wealth to children. The comparison of the old-age welfare system in Europe and that in the United States illuminates the goal of policies, or the state ideology, designed to influence individual-level wealth accumulation. Although the state is often viewed as the safety net for older people in developed countries, increasingly many Americans are turning to family for support as they are entering the third and fourth ages without any private wealth and substantial assets. Both economic and sociocultural variables must be considered if an understanding of norms governing gift-giving behavior and inheritance practice is to be achieved. In Chapter 4, I extend this discussion, presenting a theoretical model of nonfinancial factors influencing gift giving and detailing views of how we think about wealth in our lives. Financial security depends on myriad factors and the chapter analyzes facets of the moral dimensions of gift giving that embody core family values.

CHAPTER FOUR

Dimensions of Giving between Generations

Should not the giver be thankful that the receiver received? Is not giving a need? Is not receiving, mercy?

—*Friedrich W. Nietzsche (1844–1900)*

Today, there are essentially two methods of transferring wealth from one generation to the next: gift giving and inheritance. In the former, a living relative gives a cash grant to a specific person. This in effect distributes the recipient's inheritance before the donor actually dies. The second method is the traditional will, which takes effect upon a person's death and instructs the executor of the will in how chosen people or organizations will inherit the estate. Whether the exchanges occur before or after one's death, it is clear that the transfer of wealth, including the intentions, motivations, and gratitude behind decision-making processes related to gift and estate transfers, is a two-way street. The donor views the exchange out of concern for both the needs and preferences of the entire family—that is, the donor (the parent) and the recipient (the child or grandchild).

Experts suggest that older adults are motivated to pass on wealth for a host of reasons, not the least of which is predicated on the assumption that the fate of others must be weighed against that of the donor's preference and desire to give. Decisions over money often are not rational, however. If not discussed and properly managed, financial matters are fraught with potential peril and can tear families apart. Often emotionally charged, family financial decisions can cause tremendous friction between parents and adult children. Aside from social psychological factors and family household experiences, external factors such as estate taxes affect bequest motives (Kopczuk and Slemrod, 2003), though research shows that less than 5 percent of heirs, amounting to 98,000 adults age 20 and older, filed estate tax returns in 1998 (Hoyert, Kochanek, and Murphy, 1999). The following explains the complex context in which gift giving and inheritance decisions are made. Rationality and reason often play little part in how money is distributed, as is made apparent. Emotions and memories, good and bad, are often the driving forces in bequests.

THE JOY OF GIVING

While significant demographic and policy trends allow for intergenerational transfers of various types, including material and nonmonetary flows over the extended life course, economic exchanges are also shaped by particular characteristics within and between families. Material exchanges and their relation to health, education, and welfare needs, as well as cultural values toward filial expectations and responsibility, affect the types of help received from and given to family members (Groger and Kunkel, 1995). In our utilitarian society, we think of money as just money. At first sight, the gift seems to be free, spontaneous, and voluntary, but it is much more than a simple economic commodity exchange (Hyde, 1983). Cultural anthropologists have shown that in traditional societies gift giving is a deeply moral as well as economic act (Graeber, 2001). The exchange of gifts and the elaborate rules governing it define status and power, and they differentiate kin from nonkin. Gifts also impose obligations of reciprocity that bind one individual or group to another, further defining their relationships.

French sociologist Marcel Mauss (1990) argues that the motives behind gift giving and inheritance are as complicated today as they were in the past. He believes that gifts have always taken on special meaning and are not simply acts of good will, that giving money is not merely an economic act. He identified three types of obligations associated with gift exchanges: giving, receiving, and reciprocity.

In discussing the Maori spirit of gift exchange he says, "They had a kind of exchange system, or rather one of giving presents that must ultimately either be reciprocated or given back" (p. 10). In Polynesian society, the Maori principle of gift giving is guided by the idea of *mana*, which refers to the moral source of authority and prestige derived from the wealth emblematic in the reciprocal nature of gift exchange. By this principle, one must give gifts in order to maintain and increase *mana*, and one reciprocates in order to prevent oneself from losing it.

The obligations to give and to allow reciprocation were paramount because reject-ing a gift could lead to impoverished and strained social ties. Initially, Mauss states that to do so would be "to reject the bond of alliance and commonality" (p. 13). To reject such an important bond in a society that so heavily values communal identity is "tantamount to declaring war" (p. 13).

Mauss contends that in all societies gifts are embedded in social and symbolic systems of reciprocity that are supposed to be voluntary but are actually obligatory (Mauss, 1990). He assumes that forms of systematic exchange in "gift economies" are largely based on cultural norms and ethical implications of giving, which ultimately depend on the interpretation of what that gift means to the relation-ship. According to Graeber, the reality of the practice of gift giving in the United States is that one often feels obligated to reciprocate in kind and, if unable to do so, may take on a moral inferiority complex. It is this sort of variation in the moral conduct that helps to explain family gift-giving practices in terms of what is morally acceptable in the context of tax and legal structures.

Sociologists are also bridging the dimension of moral values to economics (Etzioni, 1988; Zelizer, 1997). The exchange of gifts and the elaborate and implicit norms and rules governing it define status and power, and they differentiate kin from nonkin (Lévi-Strauss, 1969). Polanyi, in his most famous monograph, *The Great Transformation* (1944), wrote that a basic form of social integration is reci-procity through gift exchanges. Gifts impose obligations of reciprocity and, so-ciologists believe, bind one individual or group to another, further defining their relationships (Douglas, 1990; Polanyi, 1944; Lévi-Strauss, 1969). Contemporary exchanges, then, are governed by implicit rules that define the relationship be-tween people. Often, families managing money in late life make what appears to an attorney to be an irrational choice—for example, disinheriting a son because he married someone of a different social class. Because of family culture, the decision of an older parent to act against an adult child may be quite logical and an instrumental act in light of a parent's desire to uphold those beliefs. In the absence of clearly established social norms for intergenerational exchanges, especially before death, what accounts for differences in the quality of relations between parents and their adult children?

Many of us have experienced what gift exchanges involve and how they work. In my research, we found many instances which are described in great detail in Chapters 5 and 6. One that warrants mentioning here, though, is an extreme example and a sad story of the complexity of gift exchanges experienced by many elderly loved ones on the cusp of needing assistance with daily life. For frail and infirm aging parents, the expectations of adult children to provide family elder care in exchange for the years of financial support is fraught with mixed emotions. Consider Gloria Torres, a middle-class Latina in the throes of midlife. She loves her mother, Mrs. Vargas, now in her early eighties, and has received many early transfers from her, including a college education from a leading state university. Although she has an "empty nest"—her only son, in his midtwenties, lives elsewhere—she is ambivalent about having her mother move in to her household with her husband if Mrs. Vargas has a serious decline in health. Emotionally, it is a difficult issue. She confides that she tries not to think about it because she is terrified of what she would need to do if something happened to her mother, like if she fell and broke her hip. "As time goes by, nobody in the world matters more to me than my husband and I am not prepared to sacrifice him for my mother." Her husband shares that same concern. He recognizes, however, that his mother-in-law would find it problematic to cover the cost of long-term care in either an assisted living facility or personal care home. This expenditure would also reduce the amount that Gloria's mother would be able to bequeath to her and her sister, Ana. For both sisters, the inheritance is not large enough for them to retire on, but for Ana, the money could help get her out of debt.

The siblings had spoken little about the dilemma until the dreaded event happened. Mrs. Vargas fell and was hospitalized for a broken hip, a fairly typical event among elderly women. She was discharged from a hospital to a nursing facility for rehabilitation from hip surgery and was finally discharged to her home, but she needs home health care, which will be provided by Medicare for 100 days. The main problem is that after the 100 days are past, she will still require some help with managing her blood sugars, preparing meals, housekeeping, and transportation, but Gloria and her sister work full time and are unable to provide the amount and level of assistance required in the long term. Plus, Gloria has recently been diagnosed with advanced breast cancer and must deal with her own health crisis. While Ana adores her mother, the reality is that, as a divorced 55-year-old woman with major credit card debt and student loans, she has no capacity to shoulder the burden alone. She is working two jobs and trying to make ends meet herself.

This is a prototypical example; aging parents don't "plan to fail," but they fail to plan for their health needs and retirement. Even for a modest inheritance, planning for long-term care financing can be the firewall to protect their nest egg and family stability. However, inheritances are not a significant issue in retirement planning for many parents, especially aging Baby Boomers. More often than not, a family discussion of who will be leaving money to whom and how much doesn't happen at any time during the life course. Perhaps the saddest family circumstances involve the animosity that develops between siblings when one sibling ends up carrying most of the caregiving burden for elderly parents. And, while most parents would never want to contribute to that situation, it happens quite often.

As the Silent Generation of elderly parents is living longer and suffering declining health, research shows they will spend down their assets faster than previous generations, leaving many Baby Boomers without any inheritance (see Munnell et al., 2003). Many adult children may find that they are left to bail out themselves. For late-life families, what this means is that communicating about estate planning is crucial for lasting family harmony. But what does this actually involve? The process is complicated by the fact that gift-giving behaviors result in part from what I term "family ideologies" concerning money and other material exchanges. The term "ideology" reflects the fact that attitudes about money and how it should be shared among family members are part of larger belief systems concerning who owes what to whom and what one generation can expect from another. Such beliefs are often passed from one generation to the next. On the other hand, one's own experiences with earning, saving, and spending, as well as one's own personality, also affect one's attitudes about money.

Differences in gift giving within the family are influenced by more than just ideology, though. They also reflect the intensity and emotional content of family members' interactions. They are often colored by the past and by life events, such as divorce, that happened long ago or by problems that persist into the present. It has also been shown that adult children who receive assistance tend to be younger, to be unmarried, to have children, and to have completed less schooling, and that parents who give assistance tend to be better off in terms of income, wealth, and education. Conversely, widowed and divorced parents do not provide as much support to their children (see Lye, 1996, for a review). Other research shows that children who spend more time in shared activities with their aging mothers and fathers tend to receive greater financial supports from their parents before death (Silverstein et al., 2002). Silverstein and colleagues developed several growth curve models in the University of Southern California Longitudinal Study of Generations, to test two competing hypotheses about long-term intergenerational exchange. In the resulting statistical model, they calculate average rates of change in social support provided to elderly parents between 1985 and 1997 and consider whether motivations for intergenerational exchanges tend to be a result of an elderly parent's emotional investment, as opposed to a financial investment, in their adult children's well-being. The analyses controlled for early parental transfers of affection, association, and tangible resources to identify the mechanism of long-term intergenerational exchange. The study offers concrete evidence of the idea that early family experiences, defined by shared social activities, have positive effects on both emotional and financial exchanges. These emotional and financial exchanges are "guided by an implicit social contract that ensures long-term reciprocity" (Silverstein et al., 2002, p. 12). This sort of emotional bond strengthens reciprocity between parent and child relationships in late life and fosters financial intergenerational exchange. The quid pro quo can be seen as an investment strategy by aging parents. As discussed in Chapter 2, generational status marked by life-altering historical events, such as the Great Depression, also influences the meaning of money in general and the propensity toward giving.

This chapter reviews important individual-level factors that influence patterns of gift giving and inheritance, and discusses the potential effects of group differences in acts of material aid. Scant evidence exists of the role of material exchanges in defining the moral tie between generations and how such financial transfers vary with other social factors. What roles, if any, do race, class, gender, and religion play in gift giving? Although there is mounting evidence that minority families have special challenges in caring for their children early in life, little is known about what happens in these families later. It is important to ask, When do financial obligations end?

THEORETICAL PERSPECTIVES ON MONEY: GOOD VERSUS EVIL?

Classic social theorists such as Marx and Weber wrote passionately about the role of money in people's lives (McClellan, 1979). They adopted a macro-level, political approach for explaining the notion of money within the inner workings of a market economy. In a section of Marx's *Economic and Philosophic Manuscripts of 1844*, the alienating power of money is described by drawing from Shakespeare and other notable philosophers:

> If money is the bond which ties me to human life and society to me, which links me to nature and to man, is money not the bond of all bonds? Can it not bind and loose all bonds? Is it therefore not the universal means of separation? It is the true agent of separation and the true cementing agent, it is the chemical power of society. (Tucker, 1978, p. 103)

In Marx's critique of capitalism, the pure value of money lies in its alienating qualities, which can transform one's individual needs and sense of self, mediating an individual's life, and creating an estranged human existence. If money is the link between people, which ties one to human life and society, then in Marxist economics, money gives way to political power (Burawoy, 2000). By having power over others, by being able to buy everything, including human labor, and by having excess funds, money reflects an *object* of eminent possession. Marx believed that a worker's product does not involve a simple transaction or a particular use but is assigned a monetary value that distorts its real meaning. The act of material exchange in and of itself is omnipotent.

Like his predecessor, Max Weber also reflected on issues at the intersection of sociology, economics, and political science, although he devoted scant attention to monetary theory. About his *Economy and Society* treatise, Maclachlan (2003) notes that Weber's treatment of financial matters is cryptic and detailed in fewer than forty pages. Weber believed that within his theoretical construction of money, unlike those often assumed by economists, the state plays a crucial role. The ontological aspects of money focused on class relations, the bureaucratic organizations, and the law as opposed to the institution of the family. The latter entity was never expounded on by either Weber or Marx. Put simply, Weber examined money only in political terms without ever discussing its influence on the family.

Another German philosopher, Georg Simmel, believed that money establishes relationships and ties people to one another by the flow of goods and services (Simmel, 1964). In his eyes, the substantive value of money was less important than its symbolic aspects. Simmel argues in fact that money is an instrument entering into nearly every social interaction and that it ultimately determines the quantity and quality of relationships that are established. Thus, unlike his colleagues, he maintains that money is an impersonal instrument. It impoverishes social life by changing the social fabric of human connections from one in which exchanges are perceived solely in terms of their monetary value to relating money to subjective values of exchange relations engendered by individuals in modern society (Deflem, 2003). Coming in the twentieth century, Simmel's perspective buttressed and extended the work of his predecessors by conceptualizing money as both a rational and a calculated act (social engagement) that ultimately depersonalized all interactions. Conceptions of gift giving and money exchange in the modern world have moved beyond a good versus evil perspective and have attracted attention from anthropologists and sociologists.

CONTEMPORARY STUDIES OF MONEY

The various interpretations and meanings of money have experienced a renewed interest in sociological inquiry. Rather than viewing money as objective and as a "means to an end," sociologists are reaching beyond these conventional notions to conceive of money as a subjective experience as opposed to a rational act, per se. Viviana Zelizer, in her innovative analysis of the social meanings of money, has brought a fresh, new sociological approach to understanding the subjective assessments of how we think about and use money (Zelizer, 1997). Going beyond early classic economic thinkers who viewed money as having unlimited force in and of itself to determine decision, she points to the fact that it is the relative importance that people attach to monetary values which gives *real* meaning to one's life and differentiates social relationships (Zelizer, 1996). When it comes to family and other social relationships, the principle is quite clear. She cites, for example, the custom that a husband does not tip his wife, as well as the practice of not offering a gift of money to a policeman because it is considered a bribe (Zelizer, 1998). In her opinion, to make such improper monetary transfers would challenge our core definitions of what those social relations entail.

Zelizer and other researchers examine this theory as it applies to social institutions like the family. Studies of intergenerational exchanges of material aid within the family have shown that several factors shape the decision-making process (Silverstein et al., 2002). The nature of giving money and gifts is largely affected by the availability of financial resources to distribute. Families with limited incomes and few assets are simply unable to give large pecuniary gifts, although gifts of small amounts of money are not unusual.

GIFTS AS ASSISTANCE

Numerous hypotheses have been proposed to explain the inheritance and gift giving differences that exist between racial and ethnic groups. Differences in family economic support among ethnic groups in later life have been linked to social class. One study documented a greater likelihood of white households' receiving an inheritance than black households. Controlling for other factors that contribute to racial differences in passing wealth to children, the data show that financial inheritance may account for between 10 percent and 20 percent of the average difference in black and white household wealth (Menchik and Jianakoplos, 1997).

The lower level of financial assistance given by older Mexican American parents may be due to the relatively greater fertility of the Hispanic population when compared to non-Hispanic whites. Some studies have found that elderly Mexican Americans tend to give less assistance to each adult child when compared to non-Hispanic whites because they have to distribute their help among a greater number of offspring (Hogan, Eggebeen, and Clogg, 1993). Put simply, latter-born siblings have to compete with their older siblings for the same pot of money. That is, younger siblings often have to wrestle their share of the estate from their older siblings.

At the same time, studies indicate that in large part, adult Hispanic children often provide support to their elderly parents. Hispanic families of all ancestral backgrounds live with their adult children to cope with chronic poverty (Angel and Tienda, 1982). Numerous studies point out that coresidence between elderly parents and adult children is more often the result of economic deprivation than a special desire for that arrangement. Paz and Aleman (1998) state that among the Yaquis, an indigenous group that migrated from Sonora Mexico to Arizona at the beginning of the twentieth century, the predominant reason for elders to live with their adult children is the need for a decent quality of life. The Yaquis they studied were so poor and possessed so few economic resources that living together was the best way to cope with their dire economic straits. Some research suggests that if elderly Hispanic Americans were given the opportunity and had the economic resources, most would choose to live in their own home rather than with their children (De Vos and Arias, 2001).

Here we begin to see a racial and ethnic difference in giving patterns, even among similar economic classes. A minister mentions in a sermon delivered several years ago that she personally observed the reciprocity of nonpecuniary gifts and its impact on the quality of interpersonal relations. She states:

> In my old neighborhood in Chicago, I lived right next door to a seamstress who worked out of her tiny apartment. She was single with grown children and one school-aged son. Puerto Rican, she struggled with English and never had enough money. She often didn't have enough money to have her phone hooked up. And yet she lived in the gift-based economy. . . . Although she rarely had money to cook other than rice and beans for a meal (the only meal usually), once a month or more she would show up on my doorstep with a bowl of rice. "I made too much" she would say, or "I have extra today." She knew my son Peter loved her rice, and she enjoyed sharing. But after the second time she brought rice, I felt the obligation of her gift-based society. I knew that every so often, I needed to make too much, or have a little extra. And I did. In that way, we built a friendship, and she varied her diet a bit from the rice and beans. At first, my mind had a difficult time with feeling the obligation this woman was pulling me into. Later my heart knew that she was artfully building a relationship with skills she had learned from childhood which nurtured and sustained us both through many trials. (Hochgraf, 1999, p. 3)

African American and Latino families, for example, give less financial assistance to adult children than non-Hispanic white families (Hogan, Eggebeen, and

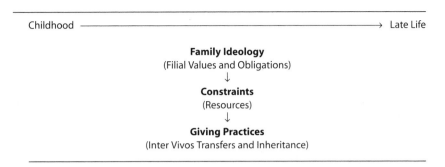

Figure 4.1. Contextual Model of Gift Giving in Late Life

Clogg, 1993; Jayakody, 1998; Lee and Aytac, 1998; Rosenzweig and Wolpin, 1993; Silverstein and Waite, 1993; Wong, Capoferro, and Soldo, 1999). Blacks give half of what white parents give to their children. Goldscheider and Goldscheider (1991) report that blacks invest less in their children's college education, regardless of their economic situation. In a recent in-depth study of 200 families in Los Angeles, St. Louis, and Boston, Shapiro (2003) illustrates that fundamental racial inequalities persist in America, not as a result of the income gap, but because African Americans have not benefited as much as whites from intergenerational wealth transfers. It is often the financial help from their middle-class white parents, for example, that enables white Americans to purchase their first home, giving them a substantial head start in their adult life (Shapiro, 2003). Some researchers contend that Hispanic parents give more than they receive and that Latino children tend to not help their parents even though they may need it (Dietz, 1995).

The model in Figure 4.1 depicts countervailing forces that account for differences in gift giving. What really explains the reciprocal nature of support are structural factors (i.e., resources), and in the case of children's gifts to parents, it is closely linked to major life events, such as eldercare giving (Henretta et al., 1997; Soldo, Wolf, and Agree, 1990; Stoller, 1983; Talbott, 1990), income need (Angel, Angel, McClellan, and Markides, 1996; Angel, Angel, Lee, and Markides, 1999), and housing assistance (Crimmins and Ingegneri, 1990). The model treats a parent's declining health or income as a constraint on the frequency and amount of giving.

In addition, in this model the concept of filial piety, meaning the correct way adult children should act toward their parents, may affect the quality of intergenerational relations (i.e., the degree of solidarity within the relationship) and, as a result, the extent of financial gifts, material aid, and bequests. Namely, norms of filial expectation, what elders desire from their children, and perceptions of filial obligations or responsibilities, what children think they should receive from their elderly parents, vary by the amount of financial resources available in families, as well as norms of obligation. Many adult children feel that gifts from their parents are made and received out of love, and these gifts occur throughout their adult lives. It provides the foundation of a family's ideology, and the moral dimensions for all attitudes of how a parent feels toward their child. If an elderly parent lacks moral authority, for example, an adult child may feel less obligated or inclined to take care of the parent, to visit frequently, and to show love, respect, and support. This moral conduct, in turn, may reduce an elderly parent's sense of obligation to provide money and material aid, even during a child's need of support as the result of divorce, widowhood, bankruptcy, or other stressful life event. Thus, taken together, the quality of elders' attitude (affect) toward their children, the opportunity for exchange, and a child's request for assistance, such as financial advice on how to care for a grandchild with special health care needs, profoundly affect reciprocity across generations.

Generational status may affect these norms of filial expectation and perceptions of filial obligation. Many elderly Americans in the Silent Generation believe that their children should be indebted to them; consequently, they expect to receive some type of instrumental aid from their children in the event of poor health, especially if they lose executive function, the ability to make decisions about financial matters. A mother who loses her husband and has a meager retirement income may believe that her children are obligated to provide housing assistance or financial assistance in addition to money management activities like help with filing a tax return, paying medical bills, and budgeting. Adults born between 1946 and 1964, the cohort now known as the Baby Boomers, on the other hand, have different experiences, values, and expectations from previous cohorts. They are healthier, wealthier, and living longer than their parents. They express greater confidence and a desire for independence. And, while a majority of workers on the verge of retirement voice concerns about whether they will have enough money for a secure retirement given the financial hardship suffered as a result of excess debt or a realistic concern about the cost of health care, housing, and energy, they nonetheless have developed a taste for privacy, control over their own daily routines, and options to enjoy the fruits of their labor. That identity, emblematic of the Baby Boomer cohort, will shape their overwhelming desire to oversee their financial future and will be reflected in both consumption patterns and work behavior.

Therefore, generational status has a dual effect on gift giving in later life in that it affects both the amount of financial resources available in a particular family as well as cultural norms of obligation. The model above, I argue, addresses how economic constraints alone do not ultimately determine the underlying motivation of an intergenerational transaction. Many adult children believe that when they receive gifts from their parents it is because the parents love them. The act itself is viewed as an unconditional love, seen as infinite and measureless. An appreciation of filial piety or family ideology may lead one to discover alternative explanations. The literature reviewed in the remainder of this chapter suggests that this may be the case. It also lays the foundation for the narrative analyses that will be presented in Chapters 5 and 6.

CONTEXTUALIZING GIFT GIVING

The first factor influencing parents' propensity to give to their adult children is harnessed in norms of filial obligations. That norms play a fundamental role in economic transfers is confirmed by other researchers examining social exchange theory; the expectations are tied to repaying debt (Homans, 1974). Molm and Cook (1995) put it this way: "Whereas classical microeconomic theory typically assumed the absence of long-term relations between exchange partners and the independence of sequential exchange transactions, social exchange theory took as its subject matter . . . the more or less enduring relations that form between specific partners" (p. 210). When parents give to their children or vice versa, it creates an obligation from which family solidarity is built (Homans, 1958). Theoretically, those feelings and expectations of mutual reciprocity provide the social glue to keep families together throughout the life course (Emerson, 1962). For instance, what is learned in childhood from the observed attitude of parents toward grandparents will affect the next generation's attitudes.

In this respect, Ribar and Wilhelm (2006) used a three-generation survey of Mexican Americans living in San Antonio, Texas, from 1989 to 1991 to analyze whether the attitudes of adult children toward their parents were transmitted and practiced by the third generation. They found that attitudes toward coresidence and financial help in younger generations were positively affected by their parents' attitudes toward their elderly parents.

Silverstein and colleagues (2002) reach a similar conclusion from their analyses of six waves of data in the University of Southern California Longitudinal Study of Generations. The sample consisted of 501 children who participated in the 1971 survey and who had at least one parent surviving in 1985. The motivation of adult children to provide social support to their aged parents is partially rooted in earlier family experiences and guided by an implicit social contract that ensures long-term reciprocity. The investigators found that receiving greater financial support from parents in 1971 raised the marginal rate at which middle-aged children provided emotional and instrumental support, thus supporting theories of reciprocity. The extent of support increased over time. On the other hand, if elderly mothers were in poor health and required assistance with activities of daily life, adult children adopted a caregiving role regardless of receiving any inter vivos transfers from their parents. The latter finding supports a theoretical model of altruism, or a nonreciprocal motivation for exchange.

SIMPLY LOVE

A related factor motivating financial transfers comes mainly from parents' feelings of affection toward their children and sentimental values. Parents want to give material gifts to their children for the simple reason that it conveys the love and appreciation they have had for them over the life course (Bengtson and Roberts, 1991). Kahn and Antonucci's (1981) social convoy model provides a framework for understanding why parents give emotional support to one another throughout their lives. In this model, close relationships with family members are viewed as continuations of early attachment relations, governed by cultural norms and past relationship experiences. This model suggests that a person is enmeshed in a number of social relationships that move with the person through time, like a train along the tracks of life. Persons in such relationships give emotional support to one another throughout their lives. Such relationships make up three circles of persons—spouses, children, and friends—whose degree of influence and provision of support for one another vary. Thus, family gift giving evolves from the parent's inner circle of relationships, such as children, and is thought to ensue from changes in age-related social norms, like college education, a first home, a new grandchild, and so on.

FELLOWSHIP FOR FUNDS

Exchanges, then, occur when both parent and child perceive a satisfactory relationship (Blieszner, 1986). Social scientists who have studied the family have noted three basic dimensions on which intergenerational relationships can be evaluated (Bengtson and Roberts, 1991). These are: (1) affinity, defined as emotional closeness and perceived agreement of opinions between generations; (2) opportunity structure, defined as frequency of contact and residential proximity between generations; and (3) functional exchange, which are flows of social support between generations.

From these three dimensions, intergenerational relations can be categorized into underlying ideal types of families, ranging from *closely knit*, defined as being connected on all three dimensions, to *estranged*, having no intergenerational connections on any dimension. The dimensions vary by gender and family type. Not surprisingly, adult children are more likely to have a tight-knit relationship with their mother than with their father, and they are more likely to have a detached relationship with their father than with their mother. Another pattern is that relationships with divorced parents, divorced fathers in particular, are more than three times more likely to be detached (Acock and Demo, 1994). Blacks report less contact with fathers after late-life divorce but more social exchange with mothers than whites (Umberson, 1992).

Hashimoto (1996) argues that the form and function of the intergenerational exchanges largely determine the quality and "symbolic equity" in the social contract. The meaning of intergenerational exchanges is extremely important in determining the *amount* of money given (Groger and Kunkel, 1995). Children who visit and call their parents more frequently tend to receive larger bequests (Bernheim, Shleifer, and Summers, 1985), although material aid and contact do not necessarily predict intergenerational intimacy (Thompson and Walker, 1984). Often parents are torn when deciding whether to make a "forgivable" loan when a child has not been responsible with the use of that money. Ongoing contact, a proxy for love and affection, is also positively related to social exchange (Hogan, Eggebeen, and Clogg, 1993) and to bequests (Bernheim, Shleifer, and Summers, 1985).

GIVING, NOT RECEIVING

Aging parents rarely receive more financial support from their children than they provide to their children. Adult children and their parents have frequent contact and emotionally satisfying relationships, but exchanges of practical and financial assistance are uncommon. Studies have shown significant differences in instrumental supports, including inter vivos transfers. But as discussed later in this chapter, this pattern has been scrutinized in recent years.

Most bequests are not accidental, and planning to give gifts before and after one's death is the result of two factors. A primary reason of passing on wealth to children is purposeful, with the ultimate decisions rooted in a desire to leave a legacy for children and grandchildren. Some studies show that bequests are independent of child behavior. To be sure, Wilhelm (1996) reported that over three-fourths of bequests made by decedents are divided equally among heirs. He used inheritance information from the federal estate tax returns of the richest people to show that rich decedents tend to bequeath equally to their children. The finding clarifies the estate division question and implies a theoretical generalization of the common assumption in the altruistic model. Lower average income of children usually does not lead to significantly larger bequests from their parents.

A second motive for bequests has to do with the *needs* of middle-aged children or elderly parents themselves. As one enters midlife, one experiences both negative and positive events that call for large expenditures (Cooney and Uhlenberg, 1992; Greenberg and Becker, 1988). Middle-class parents often assist their children with the purchasing of their first home (Mancini and Blieszner, 1989; Ward and Spitze, 1992). Langbein (1988) argues that paying for a child's education rather than transferring assets is today the characteristic model of intergenerational wealth transfers in the United States.

But gifts are also often provided in response to a family member's need for financial assistance owing to adverse life events, like divorce, debt, or illness, especially for women (Eggebeen, 1992). Today, women are less likely than men to have a retirement plan, and even when they do they receive significantly lower pensions (Wilmoth and Koso, 2002). In combination with increasing divorce rates and the fact that widowhood often results in greatly reduced income, this means that many women will find themselves in serious economic difficulties in old age (Holden and Smeeding, 1990; Holden and Kuo, 1996; Holden and Smock, 1991; Wise, 1996; Zick and Smith, 1991). This accumulation of risk is revealed in the fact that the poverty rates for men and women diverge with age (Johnson, Sambamoorthi, and Crystal, 2003). By the time they reach age 65, women are nearly twice as likely as men to have incomes below 125 percent of the poverty level (U.S. Census Bureau, 2002). Given the lifelong labor force disadvantages faced by African Americans and Latinos, such women face a particularly elevated risk of low income. Approximately one-fourth of African American and Hispanic women over 65 have incomes below 125 percent of poverty (Bound, Schoenbaum, and Waidmann, 1996).

For African American and Latino women, restricted employment opportunities and low educational levels make retirement planning irrelevant, and for many of these women marriage is no guarantee of security (Wilson, 1996). The lowered earning capacity of many African American and Latino husbands means that the married couple does not have the opportunity to accumulate assets (Crystal, Shea, and Krishnaswami, 1992). In such cases, when a husband dies he leaves his wife little wealth and no long-term financial security. For these women the problem is also compounded by the increasing risk of marital disruption earlier in life (Haider, Jacknowitz, and Schoeni, 2003). For example, Johnson and Favreault (2004) report that single mothers who spend more than ten years raising children alone are 55 percent more likely than married women with children to live in poverty postretirement. For these reasons, low-income mothers tend to rely on their parents for financial support, especially to provide the children's basic necessities and, if possible, larger gifts or loans.

At the same time, middle-aged parents may also assist both their children in young adulthood and their elderly parents. Henretta, Grundy, and Harris (2001) used data from the Health and Retirement Study (HRS) and the British Retirement Survey (BRS) to look at differences in various transfers across a broad age span of individuals, from younger to near-retirement age. The HRS represents the most comprehensive panel survey of the middle generation and is an ongoing study directed, as mentioned earlier, by researchers from the University of Michigan and funded by the National Institute on Aging (NIA). The BRS is conducted by the Office for National Statistics on behalf of the U.K. Department of Social Security.

Henretta and colleagues employed these surveys to see if there were any differences in transfer by people aged 55–63. They found that among a sample of middle-aged women, divorce tended to lead not only to greater intergenerational coresidence but also to financial transfers. Almost one out of five women aged 55 to 63 in the sandwich generation in the United States were twice as likely as those in the United Kingdom to help support a child financially (Henretta, Grundy, and Harris, 2001). In other words, British women in the midlife squeeze have fewer family demands than their American counterparts. In a global perspective of just how much a longer life expectancy will affect the potential demand for intergenerational exchanges between middle-aged women and their children and elderly parents, American women were three times as likely as middle-aged women in Great Britain to have a child and a living parent for whom they were providing financial assistance. This is an interesting finding, and it can be explained in part by the lower adult mortality among women in the United States.

Other analyses of the HRS provide empirical evidence for altruistic motives for transfers of money going to less-well-off children (McGarry and Schoeni, 1995, 1997). Contrary to the current literature on bequests, which suggests that parents give transfers equally to all children, McGarry and Schoeni found a more complex picture in terms of inter vivos transfers. Parents do not usually give when the child has no pressing need. Evidently, respondents give greater financial assistance to their less-well-off children than to their children with higher incomes. Financial transfers to the elderly parents are also found to be directly related to their needs for assistance. These results hold both for the incidence and the amounts of transfers. Such gifts buffer or protect the children from economic hardship. Thus, unequal bequests may be tied to exchange motives.

Cash assistance is another important form of support the middle generation provides. McGarry and Schoeni (1997) found that approximately one-third of adult children receive cash assistance from their middle-aged parents compared with less than one-fifth of elderly parents. Thirty percent of the middle generation's coresident adult children received transfers of $500 or more per year from their middle-aged parents. Among those who received transfers, the mean value was $4,979 in 1992 dollars. By contrast, 17 percent of the middle generation's coresident elderly parents received transfers of more than $500 per year from their middle-aged children; the mean dollar value of those transfers was $2,128.

Coresident parents and children are not the only ones receiving cash assistance from the middle generation. Fourteen percent of non-coresident adult children received transfers of $500 or more per year; the mean value was $3,061. Seven percent of the middle generation's non-coresident elderly parents received such transfers; the mean dollar value was $2,125.

Although middle-aged parents give substantially to their adult children, they do not give equally. Middle-aged parents with more than one adult child do not always give to all their adult children in a year, and if they do, they usually do not give equal amounts. The data in the present study suggest that these inequities exist because parents give more to the children who are most in need. Children who receive assistance have lower incomes. They are on average younger, less likely to own a home or to be married, and more likely to be in school. The data also suggest that parents who give are more able to do so. Parents making transfers of $500 or more are better off financially. They are also more likely to be white, educated, and have fewer children.

Grandparents sometimes cover the cost of child care (Burton and Dilworth-Anderson, 1991). The motivation to provide for caregiving of grandchildren, either in kind or financially, is to allow parents to return to their jobs. Working mothers across the economic spectrum often cannot afford day care fees, whereas most grandparents watch over their grandchildren for free or for a small payment. As a result, mothers living below the poverty level rely heavily on grandparents, the children's father, or another relative to provide child care (Smith, 2003).

Sometimes grandparents find themselves having to assume full-time care for their grandchildren. According to 1997 census data, of the 3.9 million children receiving care by grandparents, more than one-third (37 percent) were living without any parents present (Casper and Bryson, 1998). Several reasons account for grandparents adopting this role, which is often the result of an adult daughter or son's transgression. Increasing drug abuse among daughters and occasionally the drug abuse of sons, teen pregnancy, divorce, the rapid rise of single parent households, mental and physical illnesses, HIV disease and AIDS, child abuse and neglect, and incarceration are a few of the most common explanations offered (Burton, Kasper, Shore et al., 1995; Casper and Bryson, 1998; Minkler, Roe, and Price, 1992; Minkler and Roe, 1993). This situation is often fraught with economic difficulties. Because many elderly people are already living on a low income, taking on the caregiving responsibilities for a grandchild may put their economic future in jeopardy (Minkler and Roe, 1993).

Support of elders by middle-aged children may be in response to some need brought on by an emergency (Hogan and Eggebeen, 1995). This is also true for adult children whose parent has suffered a decline in the capacity to carry out necessary tasks, like grocery shopping and meal preparation (Hogan and Eggebeen, 1995). More often than not, the adult children are providing assistance with daily living to the elder, yet they do not receive money as payment or help funding the care of the elder.

Nonetheless, study after study shows that most elderly middle-class parents do not want to be a burden to their children and do not want to encumber their children's lives (Angel, 1991; Angel and Angel, 1997; Blieszner and Mancini, 1987).

Low-income families may have no choice but to be dependent on their adult children, however (Angel and Angel, 1997). For instance, as later-life immigrants of Mexican origin arrive in the United States with few assets and few opportunities or time to get a good job and to save for retirement, they depend deeply on their families to satisfy their needs. For many older Mexican Americans, their desire to rely on children for support is not only a culturally based value but also a health and economic necessity (Angel et al., 1996; Angel et al., 1999). Mexican American elders with low levels of education and assimilation have greater risks of psychological distress and cognitive functional limitations, and they tend to possess few coping mechanisms. This is just one example of how social isolation among monolingual Spanish-speakers of Mexican origin can present adult children with a potential dependency caregiver burden in terms of lost wages from work, coresidential care arrangements, and daily financial stress.

These findings were challenged by Dietz (1995). In the analyses of the 1988 National Survey of Elderly Hispanics she found that, in spite of maintaining close contact with their children, most of the Mexican American elderly requiring assistance with daily activities did not rely on their children for support. Moreover, their children did not provide any assistance to overcome the financial needs of their elderly parents.

Other researchers call into question all of the extant evidence and argue that there are few differences between the intergenerational support experienced in Mexican American and non-Hispanic white families (Berry, 2001). Race and ethnicity does not affect class giving, they contend. Markides, Martin, and Gomez (1983), for instance, found that only a small proportion of Mexican American elders relied on their children for financial support. In fact, one study revealed that elderly Hispanics were more likely to give to their children than to receive financial help from them (Dietz, 1995). It is clear that little is known about the ways in which the Hispanic family balances competing demands of caring for their own well-being while maintaining the traditional system of mutual aid and support. Some researchers contend that, as for the African American family, the Hispanic concept of "la familia," or extended family, will be challenged as increasing numbers of Latina mothers enter the workforce to provide for their families.

Transfers from middle-aged children to their elderly parents, then, appear to be based on economic ability in terms of available assets (Smith, 1997), income (Steelman and Powell, 1991) and inter vivos cash gifts (Dunn and Phillips, 1997). The evidence supports this assertion. For example, middle-aged children who transfer $500 or more to their elderly parents are better off financially while the parents they give to are worse off. These parents are less likely to own a home, more likely to be poor, more likely to be female and unmarried, and more likely to be black than white. Overall, more dollars are transferred to worse-off parents and larger transfers are made by better-off children.

The research suggests, then, that families are an important source of economic support and that they base their support decisions, at least in part, on economic ability and the need for assistance. To some degree, the middle generation acts like government entitlement programs, by buffering elderly parents and adult children against economic hardship.

THE FAMILY LIFE CYCLE AND INHERITANCE

Although middle-aged parents may give financial gifts to their adult children and elderly parents, they are not likely to receive a family inheritance (Lye, 1996). In the National Survey of Families and Households (NSFH), a large longitudinal study of intergenerational exchanges of more than 10,000 American adults conducted by the Center for Demography and Ecology at the University of Wisconsin, information was collected about financial support adult children received from their parents. Questions related to intergenerational wealth transmissions were asked of the parent about what they had given their adult child and of the children about what they had been given. Analyses indicate that the answers from the adult child's point of view may have provided a more accurate picture of what was actually received (Bumpass and Sweet, 1997). The types of support included gifts, loans, and inheritances. The inheritance questions asked of the adult child included whether they had received an inheritance in the last year, who gave them that gift, and the dollar amount of the inheritance.

The results show that the fraction of wealth transfers received by adult children is low. Frequency distributions indicate that less than 10 percent of respondents received an inheritance between the first wave of data collection and the follow-up. Forty percent received this inheritance from their parents and about 10 percent from other relatives.

Recent data suggest that most Americans over age 70 either have already or intend to write a will. The best information about the characteristics of a representative sample of older adults comes from the National Institute on Aging's 1994 Survey of Assets and Health Dynamics among the Oldest-Old (AHEAD). Information collected about the respondent's assets includes home value, real estate, transportation, business, IRA, stocks, bonds, CDs, and checking and savings accounts (Soldo, Hurd, Rodgers, and Wallace, 1997).

The analyses are based on 8,223 respondents and are weighted to reflect the population over 70 years old in the United States. As Table 4.1 shows, considerable differences occur among various groups. A person who is married, male, well educated, non-Hispanic white, Jewish, and has a high annual income and many assets is the most likely to have a will (O'Connor, 1996). Most elderly people who create wills intend to provide for spouses and children and to distribute the inheritance equally.

Disinheritance is rare; one study indicated that less than 12 percent of wills designated disinheritance of someone who otherwise would be expected to be an heir (Schwartz, 1993). That said, state laws do require that spouses leave one-third to one-half of their estate to the surviving spouse, which removes any emotional influence on how the distribution of an estate might vary by survivorship (Rosenfeld, 1979). In the AHEAD survey, the distributive preferences indicated that 89 percent of the distributions other than for spouse or for partner were provided to biological or stepchildren.

In summary, while many studies have focused on elderly parent–child relationships in general, there has not been considerable research done on the ways in

TABLE 4.1
Characteristics of Americans over Age 70 with Wills, 1994

Demographic Characteristic	Percentage in Category	Percentage with Will
Age		
70 to 75	45.2	69.0
76 to 80	26.7	69.4
81 to 85	17.4	69.8
Over 86	10.7	67.5
Household Annual Income		
$1 to $9,000	20.4	49.4
$9,001 to $16,000	24.8	67.1
$16,001 to $28,650	26.7	73.5
More than $28,650	28.1	80.9
Household Assets		
0 to $15,437	19.7	34.2
$15,438 to $73,475	23.5	63.8
$73,476 to $174,425	26.8	79.1
More than $174,425	30.0	87.2
Gender		
Male	38.0	72.2
Female	62.0	67.2
Religious Preference		
Protestant	63.4	69.8
Catholic	26.4	67.4
Jewish	4.0	76.9
Other	1.4	65.7
No preference	4.8	64.1
Race		
White	85.1	76.4
Black	10.5	29.1
Hispanic	3.8	24.1
Other	0.7	16.0
Education		
Less than high school	55.5	61.6
High school diploma	31.2	75.7
College degree	13.3	84.7
Marital/Family Status		
Married, spouse present	48.0	75.9
Married, spouse absent	1.5	66.7
Non-married couple	0.6	57.9
Divorced or separated	4.9	52.5
Widowed	41.6	64.8
Never married	3.3	51.6

Source: Adapted from O'Connor, 1996.

which cultural attitudes influence the meaning ascribed to practices associated with intergenerational monetary exchanges. It is clear from the narrative data presented in the next two chapters that gift giving within families is influenced by a complex set of interactions and emotional exchanges. If all emotional ties have been severed, gift giving may also cease. In close families, financial benefaction may be more common and the size and value of gifts may be larger. I qualify these estimates because gift giving is related to other aspects of a family's emotional interaction, but the relationship is not completely predictable. For parents to give their children gifts of money or valuable goods, they must have adequate material resources.

Whatever factors influence gift giving between generations, such exchanges represent more than simple economic acts. Research addressing intergenerational exchanges of material aid within the family has shown that several factors shape the decision-making process. In the next chapter, I explore further dimensions of the dynamics of family gift giving. To see why families consider supporting their children, and the extent to which they report that they do so, the analysis in Chapter 5 expands to uncover the nature and meaning of early memories of intergenerational financial behaviors of Americans from different social backgrounds, spanning individuals occupying upper, middle, and lower economic strata and including older adult men and women, the married or partnered, divorced and widowed, and those from major Christian denominations.

CHAPTER FIVE

Money Memories

Narratives of the Meaning of Giving and Receiving

Real generosity toward the future lies in giving all to the present.

—Albert Camus (1913–1960)

Over the past ten years, I have spoken to hundreds of people about their attitudes toward gift giving and family inheritance. In these casual conversations I have found that even individuals close to me often have a trying time expressing their feelings. It seems that articulating any opinion—strong, weak, or neutral—on matters of family finances is difficult. Money is a sensitive topic, and most researchers, including government census officials, recognize that great care has to be taken in asking questions related to a person's income and assets. For most American families, no matter what their social stratum, discussing money matters is uncomfortable. Money is a topic that parents seldom openly discuss with children, during their early life experiences and even later, once they leave the household. Nothing lays bare feelings or creates bitter acrimony as fast as discussing monetary obligations and expectations.

HISTORY LESSONS

This discomfort respondents felt toward discussing money transcends the generations discussed here: the Silent Generation, the Baby Boomers, and, to a lesser extent, Generations X and Y. Indeed, the era when respondents grew up over-

arches the entire discussion of attitudes toward money. In this study, the participants fell mainly into two generations: The Silent Generation and the Baby
Boomers. Each generation has its own opinions on money, family, and inheritance, often based on how they were raised. Family and social expectations with
respect to money are often shared between the generations but they have a few key
differences. To fully appreciate the viewpoints expressed in the interviews, an
overview of each generation is needed.

I should note that some critics may view my characterizations of the Silent
Generation, Baby Boomers, and Gens X and Y as too broad to be very meaningful,
especially given that there is so much diversity within these age categories. Although this criticism has validity, in that it may be hard to see evidence of unique
distinctions among these birth cohorts' thinking about money, what is abundantly
clear from the data analyses that follow is the general age-graded influences on
perceptions of wealth by aged parents and adult offspring. The bottom line is that
money is earned twice; once by the Silent Generation and then by their heirs.

There is no doubt that the experiences and demographic characteristics of the
cohorts of principal interest—Baby Boomer and Silent generations—differ not
only from those of previous generations, but also from each other (Hess and
Waring, 1978). This intercohort differentiation could affect how certain groups
within birth cohorts interpret their money memories and, in turn, their expectations of inheritance.

THE SILENT GENERATION

For many older Americans, the Great Depression had a permanent impact on
the way they handle their finances. That life-altering period, when almost one-
quarter of working-age adults were unemployed and thousands of banks closed,
gave rise to massive feelings of insecurity and a grassroots movement in support of
an old-age pension. Before the landmark social insurance legislation proposed by
President Roosevelt, senior advocacy organizations, such as the Townsendites,
sought support for proposals to offer relief to elderly Americans (Amenta, 2006).
Sufficient support was not obtained for a plan which would have provided a
pension worth $200 per month to every retiree age 60 or older (Mitchell, 2000).
Nonetheless, this movement created a powerful force in both state and national
politics and contributed to the birth of the Social Security Act in 1935. If it had not
been for the aging-advocacy groups, such as the Townsend movement, middle-
class Americans might not feel the way they do today about their financial security.

These elders, dubbed the "Silent Generation," were born between 1925 and

1942 and witnessed how the absence of money can affect lives. There was not a family in America that was not affected by the Depression, in one way or another. Although they were quite young during this time, the Silents were taught or came to understand that money is never to be taken for granted. If there was money in the house, it was used to buy basic needs.

As the narratives here will indicate, most of this generation defines basic needs as food, shelter, and practical clothing. This is because they lived through a common experience of being or knowing of persons who lacked these necessities. The collective experience left indelible marks on their attitudes toward money, and also on the expectations of family.

Once the Depression was over, this generation wasted no time in reflection or self-pity. They took full advantage of governmental programs and economic growth to amass the largest amounts of assets America has ever seen, and will likely see again for some time if ever. This generation learned from the past, worked hard, and avoided debt and risk. They practiced self-sacrifice, frugality, and observed family obligations. Characteristically, many Silent Generation members feel guilty for the good fortune they now enjoy. They make amends by donating to charities or helping family members who are less fortunate. To them, much was given and therefore much is expected. This attitude holds for their own children as well. Good behavior is rewarded, bad behavior is not. Defining "bad" or "good" behavior is quite often a function of generational definitions and experiences.

Unfortunately, today, after a lifetime of saving, scrimping, and investing, many in this generation find themselves in the unlikely position of dipping into their principal to pay for health care for themselves or to support someone they love.

BABY BOOMERS

While the Silent Generation's offspring, the Baby Boomers, did not undergo the life-altering historical experiences associated with the stock market crash of 1929, they share similar attitudes and behaviors toward giving and receiving gifts. Born between 1946 and 1964, Baby Boomers experienced ghosts of the Depression. Their parents hung on to the hard-won lessons of the Depression but could not deny their children the luxuries that they themselves were not able to enjoy as children. Consequently, the Baby Boomers could be considered the "spoiled children" of the Silent Generation. They tend to indulge themselves as well as their own children. They do not mind risky investments or going into debt. They came of age in the rebellious "Me First" '60s and '70s, when anything traditional was scoffed at, along with family obligations. Baby Boomers practiced a dual-track life: they supported large-scale social causes, such as feminism, ending racism, and mitigating unilateralism, while they practiced personal discovery and bent the social rules.

Although few of their parents would consider divorce, Baby Boomers embraced it as a means to personal freedom, often ignoring the social and financial consequences to their own children. Ironically, what Hughes and O'Rand (2004) observe is that the children of Baby Boomers, the so-called Generations X and Y, are quite averse to making frivolous social or personal commitments.

While much has been written maligning Baby Boomers, Hughes and O'Rand argue that it was a pivotal generation. Its members were born into a nation transformed by four years of war, and as their lives unfolded they experienced social change and responded by creating new lifestyles that set the patterns for later generations.

As the oldest Baby Boomers begin turning 60 in 2006, their future will largely be determined by what they have achieved financially. Much of what occurs in the throes of midlife will influence self-support in old age. Compared with their parents, this generation will enjoy good physical and mental health; but it has greater intragroup income inequality, according to Hughes and O'Rand (2004). One of the main reasons for this is that Baby Boomers are more likely to experience marital and work disruptions. As Baby Boomers age, they will also be more likely than their parents to divorce, remarry, and start a new family. Serial monogamy brings a whole new set of financial obligations to both men and women. Even without marital disruption, Baby Boomers may need to rethink their employment trajectory, given that it will cost more to pay for a child's college education and to help with a child's purchase of a first home than it did when their parents were making these expenditures.

Depending on personal and family expenses, wealth inequality among Baby Boomers could widen, particularly among the daughters of the middle class if marriages and work experiences fail. Divorced women without alimony and a good job history may be thrust into the low-wage service sector to make ends meet and may have little savings left over to invest in a retirement or to give their adult children (Hughes and O'Rand, 2004). A bout of disabling illness could turn into a major financial crisis without adequate disability or medical insurance. Whether mothers in this cohort will be able to turn to their children for economic support is unknown. What is clear, though, is that the breadwinner in American families like those consisting of widowed grandmother, divorced adult daughter, and grandchild may experience a midlife financial squeeze in which financial needs exceed capacity, and that earner will be unable to help her or his parent or child.

This income insufficiency scenario could extend to older ages, resulting in fewer financial gifts and wealth passed on to children.

EXPANDING OBLIGATIONS EQUAL SHRINKING INHERITANCES

Even as one generation is tied to the other, the differences in social and familial expectations can be quite large and have lasting impacts. While the parental roles and responsibilities toward rearing a child legally end at age 18, the transmission of gifts and inheritance continues long after the child has become a grown adult (Hogan, Eggebeen, and Clogg, 1993).

Bequeathing one's estate, no matter how small, is an act of familial affirmation. It signifies love and respect for the recipients. Likewise, when inheritance is withheld because a violation of a family norm has occurred, it is as if the deceased is shunning the one who caused displeasure or shame.

Even so, outside forces sometimes wreak havoc on an elder's desire or ability to leave any estate at all. There are three fundamental challenges to bequeathing inheritances today. These are (1) a shrinking inheritance fund as seniors find their assets reduced by debt, bad investments, family obligations, health care costs, or a desire to fulfill personal goals; (2) poor inheritance planning that leaves inadequate or no instructions; and (3) family conflict and disagreements.

While routine gifts involving money during a person's lifetime may be a sticky issue, disagreements over inheritances, whether they become known before or after a loved one's death, can be heartbreaking. People often are not advised about the best way to transmit their wealth to their heirs. Disputes can result in a permanent schism among siblings and create ill will in other family members. As discussed in Chapter 1, the problem of how an older parent intends to pass down his or her assets will increasingly become a sensitive issue, for Boomers' parents are expected to bequeath several trillion dollars over the coming decades. And even though the percentage of Baby Boomers who report that they received inheritance money has remained relatively stable in recent years, fewer expect it in the future. Federal Reserve analyses of the Survey of Consumer Finances between 1989 and 1998 show that the proportion of general wealth transfers declined from 23.1 percent to 20.3 percent of U.S. households (Wolff, 2003). Employing the Federal Reserve data, researchers found that about 18 percent of children born between 1946 and 1964 reported receiving an inheritance in 2004 (AARP, 2005); the median amount was $48,000 The most likely Baby Boomers in this situation were already financially secure, defined in terms of Baby Boomer households with net worth of at least $140,000. The average amount of inheritance received by these Baby Boomer families was approximately $47,909 (Gist, 2006).

Changing expectations about whether inheritance will play a large role in retirement security rest on the assumption that Depression era parents will be living longer and needing to spend more money to support themselves, both physically and financially, in old age. To be sure, Gist and Figueiredo (2006) found in a recent survey that almost one-half (46%) of older adults interviewed stated that they felt it was important to leave an inheritance or legacy to their children, yet the majority of the Silent Generation's children are expected to make it on their own financially and not to count on receiving any inheritance. Gist's 2006 survey also reveals that about one in four respondents predicts the next generation will be worse off in retirement than they are today. Although many Baby Boomers will not count on an inheritance because they state they prefer it that way, others may not be so lucky as not to need an inheritance. Current declines in private pension coverage and the general lack of retirement financing could spell trouble on the horizon.

In addition, those who expect to leave an estate are leaving less than they had expected to (Gokhale and Kotlikoff, 2000). Likewise, the proportion of elderly people who believe it is important to leave an estate to a child after their death declined from 55.5 percent in 1992 to 46.8 percent in 1998 (AARP, 1999). Many older parents are instead drawing down their capital and passing on their wealth before their death, making an inter vivos transfer to their children or are having to spend it on their health care or on amenities before they die (McGarry and Schoeni, 1997). This last scenario is remarkable, given the Silent Generation's general intense desire to avoid debt and to help their children. This trend, known as "drawing down" or "dissaving," seems to occur in specific socioeconomic groups, according to research. These groups are discussed in the following sections.

DRAWING DOWN ASSETS

For Michael Hurd (2003), the question is whether elderly people draw down their assets before they die accidentally or intentionally. What he finds is that elderly people, regardless of the number of children, are experiencing accidental or unplanned bequests. Very wealthy people have operative bequest motives. Abel (2003) concurs with this finding and contends that, in addition to any saving for the purpose of making bequests, elderly consumers may hold precautionary savings to guard against the risk of having to incur large medical or personal care expenditures later in life. Others report similar findings (e.g., Hubbard, Skinner, and Zeldes, 1995).

Part of what may be occurring is the well-established family belief by parents that they will continue to fend for themselves and will assist their children until such time as they can no longer financially or physically do so. At that time, it becomes the children's turn to care for the parent. Under the current demographic regime, however, these familial expectations may undermine the moral obligation of caring for loved ones when they are incapacitated or as they experience a changing need for assistance.

While elderly people with children may be able to engage in informal intergenerational intrafamily risk sharing, elderly people without children may not have access to such risk-sharing arrangements and thus would require larger precautionary savings than those with children. In other words, parents have made an emotional and financial investment in their children and if a major need arises in which they, the parents, need help, they are most likely receiving it. Elderly people without children or some other support network are more likely to have to purchase assistance at the end of their lives; therefore they are less likely to engage in bequests.

DECIDING TOO LATE OR NOT AT ALL

While most older Americans want to bequeath at least a portion of their assets, many families are unfamiliar with making decisions related to family finances during the post-retirement years. They do not know the fundamentals about family economics and are unprepared to make decisions that can affect the quality of family life. Basic questions about how they are going to pass down their assets and why go unanswered. Adult children often do not know the role they are expected to play in maintaining the family's values and in managing their inheritance (Gokhale and Kotlikoff, 2000).

Likewise, only seven out of every ten elderly Americans die having written a will, and even when they have done so, mistakes have sometimes been made (Stephenson, 1996). There is conventional wisdom that siblings will know what to expect and what to do and that the executor of the will is up to the task because the majority of bequests will simply be shared equally among the children (Cox, 2003). This belief is often not accurate.

FAMILY DISAGREEMENTS

Perhaps the factor that has the largest impact on bequests and inheritances is family disagreements. As shown in the narratives that follow, family disagreements can occur at any life stage and for various reasons. Many times, the major differences between the generations are highlighted when it comes time to decide who gets what and when. This can happen after a benefactor dies but also before, when inter vivos transfers are made.

During life, offspring whose behavior is not approved of or appreciated can usually fend off oral criticism from a parent, but when a will is read, the withholding of funds or assets is a final judgment.

BACKGROUND ON THE INTERVIEWS

In this chapter, I explore a broad range of financial matters with people from all walks of life and from various social strata. To do this, in-depth interviews were conducted to get a better idea of how people felt about gift giving and passing on wealth to future generations. Data were compiled from more than 1,000 hours of transcribed interviews that took place in the course of 2001 and 2002. To protect the identity and maintain the anonymity of my subjects, I refer to them only by first name. Appendix A provides a detailed description of the data and methodology of data collection and analysis. The information provides a deeply textured description of the role of material exchanges in defining the moral tie between generations. Also toward that end, the chapter addresses filial expectations concerning who should give what to whom in adult child–parent relationships and how feelings of obligation may change as people age.

Certain patterns emerged from the data collected during the interviews. While everyone's story differed in the details, the overall effects that money had on the interviewees and their families during childhood were, relatively speaking, the same. For those growing up during the Depression era, money was absolutely necessary for security and there was no free lunch. These people almost always held firmly to the connection between money and work. They would save money to purchase presents for family members, not buy them with credit. While the evidence revealed times in which economic hardship occurred during childhood years, this hardship did not, at least as self-reported, seem to undermine the quality of intergenerational relationships. Arguably, this could be a matter of selective memory and the desire to forget any painful times. Throughout the interview, respondents clearly personified an overwhelming focus on other meaningful dimensions of family life, ones not directly tied to financial aspects of gift giving.

What follows, then, are excerpts from and analyses of biographical narratives which describe symbolic aspects of the meaning attached to gift giving from the perspective of both the parent and the adult child. The analyses highlight the centrality of family ideology, which I define as the values, beliefs, and attitudes of adult children and their elderly parents, to investigate directly the ways in which individuals make sense of who owes what to whom and what is involved in expectations regarding reciprocity or gifts and bequests. Personal interviews of elderly parents are a valuable qualitative research technique for revealing the challenges they face with end-of-life planning decisions. Because it is hard to talk about money, it was difficult to discuss certain events. Even in times of trouble, the focus was not on financial crises. Many of the recollections provide a nuanced framework of what makes up a family ideology.

To glean the factors most affecting the dynamics of the way gifts and inheritance are perceived in the family, the interview covered both the positive and negative lessons learned growing up and how the family dynamic operated currently. In many cases, the narratives of gift giving personify the core connection to major social institutions and other social structures, like age relations. For example, members of the Episcopal denomination displayed a Protestant work ethic and a strong connection to the church. Guilty feelings about spending too much money were often revealed. Many active churchgoers felt that they were not pleasing God if they were spending too much on themselves. Living simply so that others might simply live was a recurring concept. The Silent Generation benefited greatly from the economic expansion following World War II, and they display attitudes entirely different from those of later birth cohorts, due to their traumatic experiences witnessing the failure of banks and family businesses. For this reason, members of the Silent Generation, having grown up with few pleasures in tumultuous times, tend to be cautious and conservative in all aspects of their lives (Torres-Gil, 1992). The qualitative evidence will reveal that self-reliance is a defining characteristic of the Silent Generation. Consequently, many individuals from this cohort have trouble spending money on themselves. Conversely, a 1998 AARP survey of members of the Baby Boom Generation showed that one-third expect a comfortable retirement and less than one-quarter of respondents believe that they will struggle to make ends meet. Although Baby Boomers on the verge of retirement are not a monolithic group, what these data underscore is that they embody characteristics of self-reliance, independence, and indulgence

(AARP, 1999). In many ways, these two generations express different expectations toward spending and saving for their own children and other needs of daily life.

How do families transfer wealth and knowledge from one generation to the next? What forms do inter vivos transfers take today versus in the past? How have changing definitions of family changed the way wealth is transferred? The interviews were revealing on these topics. Although most respondents were wary of discussing personal financial situations, their own family situations pointed to certain constants in this sensitive topic.

EARLY BEGINNINGS OF FAMILY DYNAMICS AND MONEY

Nothing to do with money is taken for granted by those who grew up during the Great Depression. The prevailing attitude among them is one of caution and care when it comes to money. Credit, debt, and risky investments are to be avoided and, interestingly, so are family members who do not appear to be well grounded or frugal.

As we will see in Chapter 6, these sentiments transcend these persons' ideals of how much to give to their own children and how much to save for retirement. For respondents in their late thirties, forties, and fifties, memories involved with giving or receiving money were very positive. The values ascribed by adults of the Depression era, one of which was "try to live within your means," appear to have been passed on to their children. If there was something the child wanted, then the child needed to save for it. Bills and basic living expenses come first, and then if money is left over, one can have fun. Arguably, the latter expectation is consistent with conventional wisdom. Even so, the Baby Boomer generation has been portrayed by the media as more self-indulgent than their parents' generation (AARP, 1999). These narratives suggest otherwise, however.

MONEY AS A GIFT

What we have learned thus far is that a confluence of factors affects attitudes toward family wealth and retirement, including demographic characteristics, economic constraints, and generational beliefs or preferences. The quality of family relations is defined in terms of the degree to which family members report feeling close to each other, a term often labeled as "filial affinity" and which is discussed in Chapter 4.

Family ideology is a value or belief shared by kin that influences the choice of giving or not giving, making it consistent with the family's norms and obligations. Expectations in inter vivos transfers and inheritance, on the other hand, refer to a financial act or an exchange that is likely to happen. To develop a deeper understanding of how family values or ideology and expectations interact with generational effects, interviewees were first asked about the types of gifts their parents gave them when they were growing up. Holidays were special occasions, and the gift exchange reinforced the occasion's significance in the interviewees' recollections. Respondents, male and female and of all ethnic groups, repeatedly spoke about the presents they received for Christmas and birthdays. They emphasized the unpractical nature of gifts when they were younger, such as candy, and the practical things, such as clothes for special occasions, when they reached adolescence. Steve, an older man who grew up in a divorced family on a farm in Georgia, vividly remembered that his Christmas stockings were filled with hard candy, nuts, and oranges. He recalled that when he was eight years old, he and his siblings got a traditional model Lionel train. By the time he reached seventh grade his father splurged for a bicycle, so he could ride to school and sell newspapers on weekends.

Gifts of money came later on in a child's life, when personal needs were greater. Early on, toys and small presents were mentioned by respondents across all social classes and in low-, middle-, and upper-income households. David, a Baby Boomer in his late forties, recalled that birthdays were special days in his family. "When we were young, I wanted a Snoopy watch, and I received it. If I wanted a big ticket item I wouldn't get it." As David grew, money became the primary gift for birthdays. "As an adult, I got one dollar for each year of my age." Money was also used as an equalizer in his family. "My maternal grandmother had a set limit that she would give, although she would give a little more to my brother because she felt he was slighted by my mother." The practical nature of gifts continued when David went away to college. Indeed, the concept that special events had budgets was illustrated this way. "When I needed a typewriter for college, I got to choose one for my birthday and Christmas." While the typewriter exceeded the budget for one occasion, because it was a practical gift, his family allowed it to serve as the main gift for two occasions.

James grew up in an economically advantaged family, and their material exchanges were closely tied to that wealth. "Waking up on Christmas mornings, I received everything I had asked for. For birthdays I received chemistry sets and erector sets. They were not cheap toys."

For others, material gifts did not play an important part at any point in their lives. This was a result of financial pressure or religious beliefs. Jack stated, "The main gift I received from my parents was from my mother. It was a spiritual gift. My mother felt it was necessary to believe in the power of prayer and the need to establish a close relationship with God and Jesus Christ. And to stay in a place where you could live in such a way where you wouldn't have to face the temptations. Enjoy life, but you don't answer to me, but to Jesus. It was a defining thing in my life. My grandmother was also influential in passing this along. My dad, a machinist, worked many long hours, and gave me fishing trips." A respondent in her seventies fondly recalled: "I was a happy child but we didn't have a whole lot of money. We went to church, and my parents took me places. Some of my friends had more belongings than I did, but it didn't matter." Bill, who grew up in a poor rural area, said, "I would define gifts as education, strong faith, and stability. Education was important to me when I was growing up because my father and mother were farmers and had no formal education."

While money may not have been exchanged directly, many positive lessons about money were learned during childhood. Middle-class values regarding money were frequently mentioned. For example, Karl, the parent of a Baby Boomer, learned the following principle, which guides his life today, namely, to develop the self-discipline to spend only when you need to and to know the difference between necessity (including education) and amenities.

Growing up during the Depression also influenced opinions. Elderly parents felt that no matter how much or little they had, they were taught by their mothers and fathers to save as much as possible. Going into debt was wrong, and spending was to be done very frugally. Although money was tight, these respondents reported that they never felt deprived. Alice commented that being frugal was a way of life. "My mother taught me that money was important and you had to buy just the essential things. My mother took in a lot of hobos, she never turned away anyone. When there are 10 to 15 people to feed, money is tight when you have only $20 dollars. We ate leftovers. She didn't throw out anything. We never went hungry and were always clean. We didn't have bathroom facilities until I was a junior in college, which we managed to pay for with student loans and summer jobs."

Steve had strong feelings that influenced his childrearing practices: "We didn't have a lot, especially when we were very young. I learned to be frugal, to live within my means, don't waste anything. When other kids were begging their parents for money, I always had a little change in my pocket. My parents never had to buy my clothes for me after I turned 12. My kids called me a tightwad. I didn't give them a lot of spending money, only their allowance."

An adult child of parents who were devout Methodists espoused traditional conservative beliefs about spending and saving, that money was not easily come by, that one had to work hard for it, and that delayed gratification paid off. Nonetheless, he and his siblings did not always abide by these guiding principles. As Jack explained: "My dad was a business manager and reconciled my bank book. He didn't place a lot of personal value on money, but would help others with money problems. My mother on the other hand, was financially illiterate, and was a clothes hound. She was a little more extravagant and had expensive tastes. From my parents, I was taught to be moderate, to value quality in items, to be practical, and balanced. I did learn, too, that money was not made out of cotton and to not spend too much. I was always scolded for spending too much of my allowance."

On the other hand, another man stated: "I didn't learn to save and to be frugal. If you are smart and well educated you should be able to make a lot of money. I was not taught how to spend. My mother did not work and she spent too much money. My father had trouble handling money, and projected arrogance toward it."

MONEY WITH STRINGS ATTACHED

Weekly chores, good grades, and other behaviors were often attached to receiving an allowance. The amount was usually tied to the activity's perceived value. One gentleman described it this way: "We had a fairly modest allowance. Ten cents per grade paid weekly, with quarterly extras, like for clothing. This started around 10 or 12 years. On report card times, regardless, we got something. One-third of our money went to God, one-third was spent on things, one-third was saved." Sometimes the payment calculation was well established. The following example from a woman in her midthirties illustrates this: "I got allowance for doing various chores, for example, doing dishes. My father would pay for grades, every six weeks. Five dollars for every A, four dollars for every B, and three dollars for every C. If I got lousy grades, he wouldn't give me anything."

Very often these arrangements persisted into the teenage years. Stan stated: "They gave me money every week, probably 50 cents a week. For a quarter, we could buy a Coke, movie, popcorn, and a bus ride. During my adolescence I received more, I didn't work until I started teaching school. I also had chores but they were independent of my allowance. I would receive a bonus if I washed and dried dishes for discretionary spending. But I was supposed to put a certain amount in church and a certain amount in savings."

Other respondents stated that their parents did not believe in an allowance of any kind. John, for example, stated: "We didn't have anything. We did have chores, we didn't have allowance. My mother gave us money for the Methodist church collection. She would bake us an apple pie to make us something special. We were allowed to babysit to be able to purchase a new shirt."

Many parents expected children to work for amenities and luxuries. Sally, a child of the Depression, stated: "I never remember getting an allowance. If I really wanted something beyond basics, I would have to contribute. I was always aware that my mother worked her butt off and that I should work too. I worked on a military base beginning at 16 to pay for clothes. I opened my own jewelry business in order to travel to Greece."

Not receiving an allowance was often considered a good thing. Parents thought it better not to establish a carrot-and-stick approach in the adult-parent relationship. A middle-aged man who has received no loans from his elderly parents stated: "I didn't receive an allowance. But, if I had a need, I asked for it. During my senior year in high school, if I needed $20 I would ask my dad for it. By that time, I had bought into the conservatism. I probably cashed a check only once."

A married non-Hispanic white man living in an upper-middle-class neighborhood with two children takes this approach: "We are trying to move to a sense of independence in our two daughters, ages 14 and 16 years. They get an allowance of $100 per month. We are trying not to use money as a reward or punishment. We've never withheld money as result of poor grades."

HOW MONEY MATTERS

Overall, how did respondents describe what money meant to them? From the respondents' point of view, material aid embodies a set of values that in many cases has its origin in childhood experiences. Some described money as important to living a good life. Nonetheless, most felt that it has to be earned and respected. Many respondents who grew up in poverty during the Depression felt that money was crucial for meeting basic needs but also for learning how to share and how to give. In general, money was never a central focus of life for children of the Depression.

Henry, a retired military officer, stated: "Money is a major necessity. It is something that makes it possible to live, and so I can make my commitments." For one married professional Latina, money did not engender much meaning early in life, and consequently she never thought about retirement. She laments this fact today, especially now that she has major legal expenses resulting from a family dispute: "I wish I had grown up with the idea that I should focus on money. All I needed to do was to be happy, and not to worry about anything. As I got older, in my twenties and thirties, there were great income disparities that I observed as a journalist, and I asked myself how I could earn more money. I didn't equate money with financial freedom, then. Today money means freedom to do what I want to, and not feeling stressed."

By contrast, some respondents felt just the opposite way: An African American divorcee in her sixties said: "Money doesn't mean that much to me. I need money, but it has changed over the years, but this is due to a spiritual awakening. My dad didn't care about money, but my mother liked to spend. It dawned on me that I received money from my work, but that it was not mine to keep. The ability to give is more important than to acquire. I have enough. The money that I get, I live off only what I need, and the extra amount I give away."

Many of those who felt that it was more important to give than to receive had a religious upbringing. One Baby Boom respondent noted: "On the whole, I guess that I was not preoccupied about material things. I had a religious upbringing, and was not drawn to the value. By high school, I would do chores around the house to pay for items like cassette tapes. I didn't hang out at the mall for example. By the time I was 12 or 13, I was heavily involved in the church and in tune with messages of Christian faith and tradition. Money is only a means for providing for the necessities, but it is not high on my list of things I think about. At times, I wanted to give it away when I had more than I needed."

Women in retirement, especially widows and divorcees, felt that money brought economic security. A non-Hispanic white widow said, "To me it means security. I want to save for the future to do nice things." Money also means freedom to many people. Many upper-middle-class respondents would agree with one gentleman's description: "Money is nice to have, but it is not important. I've made a lot of money in the past, but I was not happier then. Much happiness is tied to free time. Taking away from personal time is a problem—you can't buy that time back." Alice, a recent widow in her late sixties, has similar feelings. From her perspective, "having extra money gives you flexibility."

For many single women, money is a major economic necessity. In the case of one widowed grandmother raising her grandson, the loss of income after losing her husband was a shock. Even though her investments help her to pay major expenses, her son has problems that are a large financial drain on her. She said: "I am getting a hard lesson. My husband died when he was 59 years old. I am okay, but every once in a while I splurge and take a trip. I am raising a grandchild and he is now 15 years old. We got him when he was 15 months old." An elderly parent from a divorced household wholeheartedly agrees: "I truly didn't think much about money. It wasn't until after the divorce that I thought about it."

Research indicates that an increasing number of older Americans are finding themselves deep in credit card debt or even filing for bankruptcy due to medical problems, divorce, and inadequate pensions (Sullivan, Warren, and Westbrook, 1999). Ironically, these economic plights are often the troubles of their Baby Boomer children and their grandchildren.

THE COSTS OF WEALTH

Interviewees perceived a downside to having too much money, and that perception affects financial planning today. As Raymond, a non-Hispanic white retired professional in his late sixties, stated: "When I was in seventh grade, a friend of mine asked me to help him deliver newspapers, and he split the money with me evenly. Here I was a 12-year-old boy with three to four dollars in my pocket. I remember getting strongly criticized by my parents because I did not save a dime of it. They said that I had blown the money, that I let them down, and that I had been a spendthrift. My reaction was, by God, I will never do that again. Their disappointment in me would be worse than a spanking. I have taken that childhood frugality, and have laid a religious lay over that, and now I have a doctrine of stewardship, where I am a master that entrusts a foreman with using money wisely. To waste $1,000 is a sin or $10.00. The one check on my frugality is that I tithe anything that I give outside my own personal needs. I can send money to a medical missionary in Ecuador. We give away more than $10,000 per year."

Wendy, an adult daughter from a middle-class family, said: "At times I felt my parents had the means to give more but they wouldn't give designer jeans. When I was in ninth grade, my mother would pay only a set amount for things, and anything above that was my responsibility to pay. Once I got a job, I paid for everything. They would give us money for Christmas. And, I would say, 'Just buy me one thing, I don't want just cash.' I wanted them to purchase me something."

Lucy, the retired African American divorcee of modest means, stated: "My family pretended they had more money than we actually had. My grandmother drove a Lincoln Continental. Both of my maternal grandparents lived with me. My grandmother bought a new car every couple of years. She traded them in and got a new one. My mother has had three cars in her lifetime. One of my mother's friends gave me a car. I felt really wonderful about it. You don't look a gift horse in the mouth. I've always been around people who were very giving."

For many respondents, a social stigma is attached to having too much money. One gentleman believes that this attitude prevented him from developing a clear understanding of how much should be earned. "I think I was picking up ambivalence toward money to provide security and level of prestige in the community, freedom, and nice opportunities. There were all sorts of messages, that there is not something good about money, there is a stigma. My grandfather, who I was close to, thought money was good. He wanted me to take over the family business—oil and gas business. My father made a point of not pursuing a financially rewarding career. His main concern was for me to find some constructive work."

One African American respondent, Dave, couldn't remember there being any serious problems about money in his family, yet he felt a sense of inferiority because they were the least well-off household in the neighborhood. He said that money "became a tool that I needed to purchase things, I was never anxious about it. Looking back on it, I was in a middle-class family, but we always strived for upper class. We didn't feel needy, but wanted more."

Other conflicts arose from not having a clear understanding of how the money was going to be used. Ted describes an example: "My dad thought my mother was financially illiterate. She was gainfully employed and would say it was her money. She would spend more and ask him for the rest. She would buy him gorgeous suits that he could care less about."

Not surprisingly, when conflicts erupted, open discussions about financial affairs were few and far between at family dinner conversations. Financial problems weren't discussed in front of children. Over and over again, respondents stated that the topic was never broached. Parents were not very open about money and did not talk about it and children never asked a lot of explicit questions. It was a forbidden subject. If there was a problem, the children were not aware of it.

A GUARDED SECRET

Respondents stated that as children they often sensed that money problems existed in the family. In some cases there were family rumors about money problems which, as one adult child confessed, she is still confused about. She laughed, "They must have taken them to their grave, because I didn't hear about them. I found out later that my dad used to loan family members money to keep them going."

While children may not know the particulars of a situation, they do hear the family whispers about money, exchanges, and hidden amounts. As children grow older, parents tend to open their communication about financial matters. Many Baby Boomer interviewees responded that while their own parents didn't talk to them about money so much, they are quite open with their own children. A savvy adult daughter shared this insight: "We talk about money management. We discuss dividends, what is an ethical stock to buy, and whether to buy tobacco stock and give that money to the church."

Money was seen as a powerful tool for sharing, negotiating, and control in family life for many. Today is no different, although money conversations occur in the open.

THE VALUE OF GIFTS

The Depression lingers on in the financial values of the generation who grew up during it. Today's elder in his or her seventies or older will have memories of life during the Great Depression and how gifts meant a great deal, no matter how trivial they may seem by today's standards. Again and again, both men and women in this age group commented on how special any sort of gift was when they were children. While it may not have been completely apparent how hard things were for their parents, as children they instinctively knew that their parents were stretching to make ends meet. So, a gift for Christmas or their birthday meant a great deal to them. Even the kindness of a neighbor in taking them to the movies was memorable. A typical comment was, "We never expected much, so when someone gave us something, it meant a great deal. The [monetary] value of the gift didn't matter at all." When these Depression era children had families of their own, they often lavished them with the gifts they themselves did not receive as children. Then the value of the gift became more important.

For these respondents, intergenerational giving, whether in the form of gifts, loans, or inheritance, is rooted in early childhood experiences. Those experiences may ultimately influence one's attitude toward financial planning and bequest intentions in adulthood. Many of the concerns about intergenerational gift giving expressed by these two generations dealt with uncertain adverse life-cycle events, including poor health, which would ultimately inhibit one's ability to pass on wealth. These concerns are also the product of various other circumstances, like a child's need for college tuition, a wedding, a housing down payment, and of constraints, such as financial capacity based on earnings and future rates of return on investments.

Remarkably, more than seventy-five years after the start of the Great Depression, that event continues to resonate in the attitudes and lives of those who lived through it and of their children. For respondents who were alive during that time, the lessons were frugality and charity. For their children, the parents made every effort to deny them nothing, as if they were trying to give their own children the type of childhood they themselves were never able to experience.

These narratives show that money and attitudes about money are colored by memories and experiences. They show that early family teachings and examples are powerful influences and have the ability to affect many generations into the future. With this in mind, the contemporary aspects of specific kin attitudes and behavior and their implications for private transfers from elderly parents to their adult children are discussed further in Chapter 6.

CHAPTER SIX

Contemporary Values and Beliefs regarding Intergenerational Transfers

A gift consists not in what is done or given,
but in the intention of the giver or doer.

—*Lucius Annaeus Seneca (4 BC–AD 65)*

IT ISN'T JUST MONEY

In agrarian societies, the rules surrounding gifts and bequests defined kinship and status and determined the boundaries of family and community, as discussed in Chapter 2. Today we view property and money as material goods to be bought, sold, or given away. Yet, the exchange of material goods and money is not so simple. Money and wealth in all their forms are complex symbols, and their exchange is profoundly moral because exchanges define the relationship between the giver and the recipient. In a very real sense, our emotional ties are intimately linked to material exchanges. The parent-child bond is a fundamental one, and exchanges between these two generations define our very social structure. Inheritance and intergenerational obligations go far beyond the mere passing of material possessions. This is why it is so important to uncover how age-related factors govern these exchanges, as well as their implications for income flows, for meaningful personal legacy, and for meeting societal needs.

As Chapter 5 revealed, people's attitudes regarding money are quite often established during childhood by family ideology and economic circumstances. Gifts are looked on as affirmations of affection and kinship for givers and recipients.

Inheritance is a form of gift giving that occurs at a particular point in the life course, and like all gift giving, the transfers of money and property involved often are quite suggestive of the relationship between the deceased and the recipient. Chapter 2 showed that, unlike in early America, today's laws of inheritance are based on the privileged nature of kinship ties, especially those among nuclear family members. Rules and patterns of inheritance, therefore, like gift giving more generally, define the boundaries of the family. When an older person chooses to disinherit a child, the act is tantamount to evicting the child from the family. At a basic level, the disinherited person's legitimacy has been revoked.

As part of the normal aging process, all of us gain personal knowledge of the problems inherent in the exchange of money while one is alive or upon one's death. As discussed in Chapter 5, although the topic of inter vivos transfers and inheritance is commonly not considered in a child's early years, later in life the issue may be so emotionally charged that it disables discussion among family members, if discussion had been allowed at all.

Chapter 5 showed that family cohesion is maintained through systems of ritual-ist gift exchange such as Christmas and birthday presents. Through his eth-nographic observations, Mauss, a French anthropologist, examines native and tribal societies and looks at "potlatches" as a case example (Mauss, 1990). Potlatch is a cultural tradition of native communities in the Pacific Northwest. It is a widely studied ritual in which sponsors, helped by their entourages, gave away resources and manufactured wealth while generating prestige for themselves. In these tribal societies, balanced reciprocity involves giving to more distantly related partners with the expectation of equivalent, but not necessarily immediate, exchange. This type of exchange system is common in tribal societies and has serious ramifica-tions for the relationship of trading partners. Against the established and clear expectations for giving and receiving among these tribal societies, how do every-day transfers in our own modern society compare? Is a gift among family members given without expectations? The narratives that follow illustrate just how often gifts are given and under what circumstances.

FAMILY VALUES AND IDEOLOGIES

In the absence of clearly established social norms for intergenerational ex-changes, especially before death, what accounts for differences between parents and their adult children? Gift-giving behaviors are a result of ideas and examples passed from one generation to the next. Based on family history and values, each generation develops expectations of what gifts should be passed on or received. On the other hand, one's own experiences with earning, saving, and spending, as well as one's own personality also affect one's attitudes about money. Differences in gift giving within the family also reflect the intensity and emotional content of family members' interactions. They are often colored by the past and by life events, such as a divorce or marriage, that happened long ago or by problems that persist into the present.

Chapter 5 illustrated that gift giving within families is influenced by a complex set of interactions and emotional exchanges which together affect expectations as to what is likely to happen. In order for parents to give their children gifts of money or valuable goods, they must have adequate material resources. Yet even poor parents often give relatively substantial gifts to their children, and those gifts can represent far more than what may be immediately apparent. Working-class Latino families, for instance, while struggling to make ends meet, report feeling obligated to take financial care of their elderly parents whenever the parents are unable to do so themselves. It appears there are role ambiguities, or a different family ideology and values and contradictory societal expectations for immigrant families associated with everyday decisions about gift giving, and that traditional patterns of exchanges in later life, such as from older parent to adult child, may be less common. Indeed, the obligation to care for their parents may have been instilled in these adult children when they were young, as their parents cared for grandparents or great-grandparents. Supporting one's elders, whether emotionally, financially, or both, is the ideology of many families, immigrant or not. For one son of a Hispanic immigrant family, financially helping his divorced parents is expected. He graduated college on scholarships and is doing better financially than his other siblings. They provide emotional and caregiving support to the parents, and he sends them money.

Further examples of role ambiguities occur among non-minority families as well. Health care is enabling people to live longer and more independently, but not completely so. Gifts of service and cash are often provided by children to their aging parents as a result. In addition, the precarious nature of the economy leaves many young families vulnerable. Sometimes new relationships are forged between parents and their children to meet individual needs. Sometimes these relationships are mutually beneficial; sometimes they simply benefit the recipient.

One unmarried woman in her midthirties is a good example. She moved from the South back East to live with her widowed father when her job became precarious. Her father wanted her to come home so she would be close to her family.

The father is getting close to retirement age and his health is not very good. While he never actually said, "I need your help," it was understood that her assistance would not be unwelcome. Now, the woman is able to telecommute to her job, make sure her father gets to the doctor and is well cared for, and she pays for upkeep on the house.

A similar situation, but with different family ideologies, is illustrated by a family living in the Hill Country of Texas. Due to bad investments, the patriarch of one old family found himself barely hanging on to a small estate. In his eighties, his health and financial situation were such that he could function on his own but could not maintain his property without assistance. He was unwilling to sell the land, because the price it would fetch in its current state was not what he considered its worth to be, yet he couldn't afford the repairs to bring it up in value. Moreover, the land was the only asset he had left to leave his children. The gentleman's youngest son decided that he could help. An arrangement was struck: the youngest son and his wife would move onto the place, build a separate, smaller house on the property, look after the father and pay for upkeep on the property. The father made it evident that, upon his death, the main house would be left to the son, while the extensive antique collection would be left to the daughter. When the son went over his father's will, the wording was such that, to keep the house, the son would have to pay half the estate's value to his chronically unemployed sister. The mutually beneficial situation had become an economic drain on the young couple as the money and time they had invested to maintain the property while the father was alive was not being considered equity. Upon the father's death, it would cost more money to settle the estate with the sister than if he had left it as it was before the young couple moved there. Unfortunately, the father was continuing a family ideology of helping a child more in need rather than considering the equity being invested by the son. For the son, his sister seemed to be being rewarded for opting for unemployment rather than under-employment.

LEAVING A LEGACY

An inheritance is a fundamental tie between generations, and it solidifies, in a final act, a person's place in the giver's life and emotions. Inter vivos gifts serve much the same purpose, though without the finality of a will. With each act of giving, or not giving, a family's values and ideologies are transferred from one generation to the next.

The research reported in Chapter 5 underlined the fact that respondents' assessments of experiences when they were young pinpoint the minimal extent and frequency of exchange between parents and adult children, and that most financial transfers in fact occur at certain life-course transitions, such as entering college or buying a home. Support from parents tends not to be constant across adulthood; the early forties are marked by the most dramatic decline in receipt of parental support.

Several other determinants of gift giving have been studied. Parents do not usually make monetary gifts when the child has no pressing need, and widowed and divorced parents do not provide as much support to their children as married couples do. It has also been shown that adult children who receive cash assistance tend to be younger, unmarried, with children, and to have completed less schooling. Also, parents who give assistance tend to be better off in terms of income, wealth, and education. Unless an adult child has special needs, middle- and upper-income parents want to divide equally their inter vivos transfers. For instance, when a young college graduate decided to open up a franchise clothing store, and not pursue an advanced degree, he was able to get the startup capital from his family. This young man's parents had paid for his siblings' law and medical schooling. Because he did not pursue further education, his parents gave him the money set aside for his continuing education to help start his business. Once again, whatever the factors influencing gift giving between generations, such exchanges represent more than simple economic acts.

The narratives that follow illustrate the concepts of transferring family ideology and assets across a wide range of socioeconomic strata.

TRANSFERRING ASSETS

Parents may transfer assets to their children during life and/or after death. The first, an inter vivos transfer, occurs as gifts of cash or property while the giver is alive. The second occurs in the execution of the directives in a will or, when a will is lacking, by a court's directive. Whether a parent decides to give away assets while still alive or as an inheritance is determined by several factors. Family values and moral obligations play an important role in decisions about gift giving in late life, as do economic factors, health care needs, and generation.

Although intergenerational support to children who are in midlife is not typical among American families, aging parents are likely to be involved in material exchanges with at least one adult child at some point. Estate planning is a concern primarily for the upper and middle classes, whenever estates are large enough to justify elaborate planning. Among the working class, passing on a modest estate may be less troublesome, and a simple will—or no will at all—may suffice. For the poor, passing anything on to later generations is rarely a possibility.

INTER VIVOS EXCHANGES

An overriding concept of inheritance is the centrality of the child's future and the importance of education. Many of our study respondents felt that education was the key to getting what one wanted out of life. It was important to give permanent loans so children could leave school without debt and get a foothold in society. Not surprisingly, giving money to adult children brings happiness to the giver and the recipient.

Cassie, a married woman, stated: "The gift for college education not only is what you can do to help someone, but also it makes you feel good." She remembered her own gratitude for scholarship money she had received. She made a further point: "It means more when you are able to look someone in the eye. . . . When I received $5,000 to $6,000 after my father died, I didn't know what to do with it. I can't remember what I spent it on. It seemed so unnatural. I would have appreciated it more if he had given me that money while he was alive."

Liz, a divorced woman, received assistance from an additional member of the preceding generation. "My father saw to it that I graduated from college without debt. I have the same goal for my sons. My oldest son will get $1,000 to start . . . married life. He will also get a $1,000 rebate from his college for graduating earlier. The other two children can go wherever they want to, but I will have to work hard to do this. My uncle gives me a $10,000 annual gift for each of my three boys. He created an account for them in order to purchase braces, college, and other medical expenses. I feel that he is extremely generous, and that I am not alone."

Expressing the pleasure parents can derive from financial transfers, one woman said: "When my son bought a condo, I offered $10,000 to him, but he didn't want it. I gave my children each $10,000 when my husband died five years ago. I told them just to hold on to it in case they needed it. I am glad that I am in the position to be able to do this."

For another mother, it was also important to help her children when they really needed it. "All of my children are adults and have children of their own. They have their own struggles and I have had to help them during various crises. They hated to ask for help because they have their pride. But I could always tell when things were not right and I would offer them some help."

Some inter vivos gifts have strings attached. Usually the child is exhibiting a behavior that is not condoned by the parent. "My son is living with a woman who doesn't pay her rent. He brings the situation up and wants to air it out with me. I laugh at him. He doesn't want any more financial help. He prefers not to accept any more gifts because he believes strings are attached." For this son, his mother's derisive attitude makes taking financial assistance from her too expensive.

These sorts of family dynamics, where strings were attached to a loan or inter vivos transfer, were observed in children. Theoretically, if the children were all good, they should deserve it. But if they were bad, they would need to reconsider. In the case of supporting a child's higher education, George stated: "In general, I believe it is important to loan children money, but you have to take into consideration how responsible your children are. You bring up passing grades, and we will pay for tuition and books. We paid for our daughter's graduate school, and afterward for her rent and utilities."

What happens when strings are not attached to inter vivos gifts? Parents want the best for their children because they desire that their children will do well in life. But unlike bequests, which are usually equally divided among heirs, inter vivos transfers occur as the result of a child's need and a parent's general concern to help a child with financial problems (Cox, 2003).

The attachment of strings is sometimes gendered. One Mexican American couple's son is angry with the unconditional support his parents have provided his divorced sister, who does not work. His parents purchased a home for her in their name and routinely send her checks. She lost custody of her daughter even though the parents paid hundreds of thousands of dollars to contest the decision. This situation harkens back to the chronically unemployed daughter receiving preferential treatment from her father, even at her brother's expense. What seems fair to the parents may not be to the children.

For most people, whatever fiscal transfer tradition is in their family is one that they will continue themselves. This is, of course, contingent on their belief that the tradition is "fair." Liz's example above, is a perfect example. She benefited from her father's and is benefiting from her uncle's financial practices toward her. She will, in turn, try to do the same for her sons. Cassie, on the other hand, felt that the financial gift from her deceased father would have been better appreciated had he given it to her while he was alive. She perhaps will change the tradition by giving inter vivos gifts, so that she and the recipient can both appreciate the gesture.

CHILDREN HELPING PARENTS

The occasions when money or other assistance flows from children to parents are often very specific: when health problems arise or retirement funds provide a meager existence or worse. Pride and ideologies that demand self-sufficiency often keep parents from asking for assistance from their children.

Parents from working-class and middle-class backgrounds feel strongly that they do not want to be a burden on their children. Spending within one's means and avoiding going into debt in later life are still important to them. Once again, the lessons learned during the Great Depression resonate in today's elderly people. As one woman put it, "My husband and I are living comfortably but we do not have a lot of amenities. We are living on Social Security and a small private budget. I tell my children that it is important to keep on a budget. We never have to ask our kids for help." This attitude usually suffices until a financial crisis arises.

Gay couples may be in a better position to help parents because they are less likely than married couples to have children to support, too. David said, "My partner's mother is in need of financial help. Both husband and wife rely heavily on Social Security." In this case, David and his partner provide the financial support while his partner's sister provides emotional and practical care to her parents.

Sometimes parents' needs are not recognized or acknowledged by children. Lauren, who is now in her midthirties, was surprised to learn what her parents thought they deserved and needed when Lauren's godmother bequeathed her a small inheritance. After learning of her good fortune, she was shocked to discover that her own parents felt that they deserved at least part of her inheritance. Perhaps they had experienced financial difficulties as a result of her father's retirement, despite the fact that he had a private pension and Social Security. However, Lauren didn't think her parents needed the money. She felt she needed the money more because she and her husband had two children to support. Of course, she would have had to pay an inheritance tax on any gift to her parents. Today, Lauren and her parents, who are in their late seventies, barely speak to one another and when they do, the topic of money is off-limits.

Leaving an inheritance is usually not an option for people facing economic stresses or hardship. It's a sad situation for all parties when a spouse dies and the surviving spouse, usually the wife, is without income or assets. Tricia recalled: "My husband's father left things in a mess when he died. He had invested in the stock market—high-risk funds—and lost thousands of dollars. He kept his wife uninformed about their financial situation, including lending money to a neighbor's son without her approval. Even worse, he never organized his tax or financial records. For this reason, she had no way to track what had happened to their money."

CHOOSING INHERITANCE

If inheritance is chosen over inter vivos gifts to transfer assets from one generation to the next, a whole set of issues are usually addressed. What do parents *expect* to leave their children and how do they intend to divide their estate? Issues of fairness color most decisions of inheritance. Deciding what is fair in blended families, how to distribute assets among children who have experienced various degrees of success or failure, or whether there is any money to leave at all greatly challenge family ideologies.

Not surprisingly, what the empirical evidence shows is that, in estate planning, most parents, regardless of ethnicity, think it is important to give each child an equal piece of the pie. They feel it is the right thing to do, and they are glad they are able to do this. An African American male lawyer stated: "Yes, I feel strongly about this. I would try to be equal. It is important to me, because I don't want to show favoritism. I would not try to do anything to cause them to feel that I was showing favoritism. It makes sense that in the long run it would have caused a lot of problems. It would prevent any resentment."

One couple stated: "We've talked about inheritance with our children, but not amounts. We will divide the estate into four. My biological children will get an eighth and that makes what we have divided up equally. My two step-children have money from their maternal grandmother. For personal items, we will make a personal list of items and they will draw numbers for them." This businesslike approach to coping with a blended family makes the parents feel like they are being fair to all. Whether their children will feel the same is unpredictable.

What if you wanted to leave something that no one wanted? This is the situation one couple is facing. As one father of a blended family described it: "We talk to them in general about their inheritance. We have some things that are going to my children and others to her children. We recently downsized our home and we want to pass items on to them. But they don't want them, they don't have room for them, and they don't want extra things." This is also the situation for Joan, who wants to leave her vast collection of eclectic things to her children, but her husband tells her they don't want it—that her stuff is dated. What is valuable to one generation may not be to the next.

Still, most respondents believe that the right way to handle their estate, however modest it may be, is to tell the children the reasons the parents wish to pass on their assets and what role they expect the children to play in maintaining the family's values. Making sure that all siblings are informed helps to avoid trouble after the parent has died. "My children know that I have an advanced directive and a will. It makes me feel proud that I can teach them to plan rather than to wait for a crisis," said one respondent.

There are risks associated with discussing one's will. Diane admits, "My oldest son is still upset because I didn't include his wife in my will. If he thinks he's going to get two-thirds he should forget it. When you are married it's both your money." A divorced African American mother flatly stated that she did not think it was right for her children to expect certain things from her in the way of inter vivos transfers and inheritance. As she put it, "That is my son's responsibility. He created [his debt] and the buck stops with the two of them."

Many parents stated that they did not expect certain things from their children in return for an inter vivos transfer and inheritance. Michael noted, "I would say probably not. I was given those things and I trust them to do well. I watched my parents give generously. My grandparents gave generously, and that freed up their ability to give to others. My children will be older, when they turn 18 to access this set-aside money for graduate school, first house, at a time in their life when they can really use it. I have some hopes from a value point of view. But I received the inheritance with no strings attached."

For those who inherit large amounts of money or property from parents, relatives, or nonkin, the bequest can profoundly alter both their financial situation and the nature and quality of those relationships. Smaller bequests can still have enough of an effect to generate jealousy and ill-will among heirs. These resentments can linger for years, and sometimes the distribution of an estate tears a family apart.

CHALLENGES TO FAMILY IDEOLOGIES

My research found that the main challenges for most respondents when deciding what to leave to whom were deciding when and how much to give children who were having financial problems, deciding what would be fair, the temptation to play favorites among children, and how to dispense inheritances in blended families.

In the case of a child who has not turned out as well as a parent had hoped or when a child has forsaken the family ideology, the will is the place where the parent gets the last word. As Lisa explains, "Even though she is younger, [my daughter] is the executrix of my estate, because my son is so irresponsible. My son has three children. His half of the estate is divided into fourths because that is the only way his children will be educated. Anything that he gets will be gone immediately."

Lisa continues, "My daughter will be in charge of the money for the two younger children, and an aunt and uncle for the grandchild who is living with me. The children can have the money at 18 if they are in college but at 30 if they are not in school." By carefully specifying who does what and who gets what, Lisa is using her money to ensure that her son's children will at least have a chance for either a college education or a financial boost in life. She is passing judgment on her son's behavior by cutting him out of the will, but she is showing love and concern for his children through her gifts and thoughtful arrangements.

A similar situation exists for a grandmother from the Silent Generation who does not approve of her younger daughter's husband. She plans on leaving that daughter's half of the estate in a trust for her children. Her older daughter, however, will get her share of the money outright. "My husband worked hard for his money and I don't think he would want me to give it to my son-in-law so he can buy frivolous things. If I put it into a trust, at least the money might be there when they are ready to go to college. My older daughter can take care of the money and use it for practical things. I don't have a problem giving it to her at all." This Silent Generation grandmother frowns on her Baby Boomer son-in-law for his spend-thrift ways. In her opinion, it is better to make sure that the grandchildren are provided for rather than the son-in-law. She knows she risks a family squabble over this, but she is resolute in her opinion and her decision.

Sometimes judgment is not a part of special provision for grandchildren. Many elders who can afford to do so carefully apportion their estate so that their grand-children as well as children are included. One couple is receiving land as an inheritance from the husband's parents and his children are being provided for in a trust. "We've talked to our children about the land inheritance. My parents have set up a trust for our children but they won't discuss the amount with the children."

Sometimes parents leave children assets specifically because they know they will be needed. They have decided that in order to be fair, they must consider each child's situation. "I have spoken to my children and told them what I am leaving to them, and why," declared one respondent. My homestead, I am leaving to my daughter because she is a single mother and has overcome her problems managing money and can pay the taxes." Here, a daughter's behavior that ob-viously had caused problems in the past—her inability to manage money—had been corrected satisfactorily and she was once again in good graces with her mother. In another example, an African American divorced woman believed that her gifts should not be distributed equally, that instead a particular child's needs should be considered. The distribution should depend on where the children are in life and what their needs are. She explained that her daughter needs a house as opposed to her son who just bought a house. Consequently, her daughter will get her house upon her death.

Hard feelings between siblings can arise when parents fail to discuss the property distribution, especially if it is not an even distribution. For example, Suzanna, a Latina in her midthirties, believes that while her mother had good intentions about her estate, her situation prevented a smooth probate. Her mother, a widow for many years, felt it was important to pay off her debt so she could pass on her wealth to her children. Her home was worth about $250,000 and comprised the bulk of her estate. But her plans fell apart when she became seriously ill and required intensive health care. Suzanna, the youngest of three daughters, was the primary caregiver, and she did not receive support from her two older sisters. After her mother died, the oldest sister, who was the executrix of her mother's estate, sought to exclude Suzanna from receiving any belongings from their mother's house. Tragically, a costly legal battle between the two has ensued over the distribution of the estate. Suzanna's mother failed to instruct her oldest daughter on how to distribute her belongings upon her death. As the only caregiver during her mother's illness, the special bond Suzanna felt with her mother has been denied by her sister. By excluding her from the estate, the sister is damaging Suzanna's place in the family and in her mother's legacy. Did Suzanna's mother play favorites by selecting the oldest sister to be executrix or is Suzanna's sister playing favorites with her other sister and consequently denying Suzanna part of her mother's legacy? Whatever the reasons, relations have soured among the sisters.

When family values or ideologies are not followed, judgment is often made or cemented in the contents of a will. One elderly family matriarch was severely upset and disappointed that her youngest son had married someone she considered beneath their social class. In her generation, social classes were well defined and behavior between them rigidly controlled. She stopped speaking to her son for his social transgression, believing that he had brought shame to the family. After many years of discussion with her family, who begged her to forgive this son, she finally began speaking to him again. However, after she died and her will was read, it became obvious that she had really only superficially forgiven him, for she had completely cut him out of the will. The judgment expressed by the will was final. She would not allow family money to be passed to someone who betrayed her family values. Even more tragic is the situation in which relations between quarreling family members have improved but a will written during the period of estrangement is not updated, and execution of the will digs up the bad feelings and perpetuates them.

Blended families often pose a special problem, especially when there are children from each side. Sometimes the blending works, but sometimes it doesn't. "My oldest daughter did not think she was part of the family so she is not included in the will," says one elderly gentleman. Similarly, the adopted children of one couple were never accepted into the woman's family. Gail's children were never able to prove themselves worthy of inclusion in her extended family, even when they cared for Gail after she developed a fatal neurological disease and her own sisters rarely visited. Then, Gail's family was outraged when she left her extensive estate to her adopted children. Her family believed that non-blood relatives should not inherit anything.

TO GIVE OR NOT TO GIVE, THAT IS THE QUESTION

These data suggest that it may be wiser to focus on what one's own needs will be than to try to read a crystal ball to understand children's expectations of a potential bequest. Decisions about how to structure asset transfers for an adult child with special needs can therefore be particularly vexing. To be sure, the most important thing to realize is that the parental role is carried into old age. Whether father or mother, birth parent, step-parent, or adoptive parent, part of life has been spent caring for the child, and this care in some ways continues throughout the life course, even into the parent's seventies, eighties, and nineties. People tend to bring this sense of responsibility to their estate planning and their lifetime planning.

However, some legal professionals from the National Academy of Elder Law Attorneys strongly believe that this may be the wrong focus (Farrell, 2001). A good example is the question that comes up in every estate planning interview about who will be an individual's attorney-in-fact under a power of attorney and who will be the executor of the will (Schaefer, 2000). An attorney-in-fact under a power of attorney is the person one names to act on one's behalf when a power of attorney is executed. That person takes action in one's stead and presumably for one's benefit. Many people feel that they have to name all of their children as agents to act for them under the power of attorney, rather than the one who is most capable in the area with which they are being entrusted. And parents do this even though they suspect it is inappropriate and ineffective (Schaefer, 2000) because they don't want to offend any of their children or exacerbate any sibling rivalries (Cox, 2003). The tendency to treat children equally originates from a parent's caring impulse toward them when they were five- and six-year-olds.

But this nondiscriminating assignment of responsibility may not be prudent. By the time people need a power of attorney or an executor, their children are typically in their fifties and sixties, and by that time the strengths and weaknesses of each are known. One may be good at making health care decisions. One may be good at making financial decisions. Those are two different strengths. Naming the one who is good at making health care decisions to be the person who makes financial decisions might be a recipe for disaster. As the work gets done by those children, they can come into conflict because the parent has not wisely applied their strengths.

Another precaution that should be taken is planning for the possibility that the elder may become mentally incapacitated. Elder lawyers frequently receive phone calls such as this: "My mother is now stroke-ridden. She's in the hospital and I need to get a power of attorney." A lawyer may not legally take instruction from an incapacitated person and prepare a document for that incapacitated person to sign. After a person becomes mentally incapable of decision making it is too late for that person to appoint a power of attorney or executor.

Special issues associated with children with severely disabling illness affect estate planning. Depending on the nature of the disability, developing a plan to support such a child may change what a parent wishes to leave to his or her children as they grow older and who is designated as the responsible party. Chapter 7 discusses a couple of strategies that some families are enacting to cope with this and similar situations.

It is clear from the nonquantitative research that families vary widely in their gift-giving behavior, depending on their social class, ethnicity, religion, and factors related to the timing of life-course transitions, such as divorce. Some parents plainly see money as one promising means of cementing the bonds with their children. Others, however, separate the meaning of money from emotional ties and do not give gifts to their adult children. Today, most middle-class parents provide for all or most of their children's college education, and many feel that such a gift is sufficient. Some help with the purchase of a home but view such money as a loan, perhaps even repayable at favorable interest rates.

In summary, many people express a deep desire to pass on as much wealth as they can to their children without sacrificing their own economic security in old age. These attitudes and opinions regarding financial exchanges in adulthood inform empirical research which suggests that parents allocate transfers to children on the basis of several criteria (Bernheim and Severinov, 2000). On balance, parents who have money give equally to their children upon their death. An expectation of services in return for their financial gifts was not revealed by these respondents. On the other hand, elderly parents do indicate personal concern about a child in dire need of assistance, and this often leads to greater financial support for the poorer among a couple's children. Certainly, inter vivos transfers are often dictated by a child's economic needs and are not distributed equally across the offspring. As discussed in Chapter 4, economists have documented this tendency toward inter vivos transfers and permanent loans to those children who are "liquidity constrained" (Cox, 2003).

Regarding inter vivos transfers, the size and nature of the gifts vary by socioeconomic status. The rich can better afford to transfer wealth to their children during their own lifetimes. Whether or not such transfers occur also depends on each family's ideology concerning money, gifts, and reciprocity. In Chapter 7, I discuss the influences of public policies and the law on gift giving, spending, and savings.

CHAPTER SEVEN

Leaving a Legacy

Personal Security, Family Obligations, and the State

It is better to give than to receive.

—*Acts* 20:35

This chapter looks at the body of issues that many families today face when planning their estate or long-term care. Increasingly, planning is essential; about two-thirds of Americans believe it is important to leave their heirs a bequest, but some people are perplexed by whether to spend their estate while alive or preserve wealth so it can be passed on to generations that follow (Munnell and Sundén, 2003). As noted in Chapter 6, the important social-psychological processes accounting for gift-giving motives include multidimensional constructs associated with personal and societal values regarding money and family. These values are deeply rooted in several theoretical, inextricably linked perspectives. These include general feelings of concern about the welfare of future beneficiaries, making sacrifices to help children, expected exchanges from children based on their own capacity to give and values, and quality of family life in later years. In short, there are many motives for making bequests. Feelings of financial security and values toward money and material wealth have a profound effect on successful aging and the quality of family life in the later years.

Many people are motivated to leave a legacy to others outside the immediate family. Inter vivos transfers to friends and charitable organizations are becoming a considerable portion of wealth transfers. The 1998 Survey of Consumer Finances, which looked at data for 12 million American families, reported that in 1997 they gave nearly $64 million to nonrelatives. The amounts given ranged from $20 to more than $1 million, with the average gift being $3,000 (Schervish and Havens, 2003).

In addition to social-psychological processes that influence giving, governmental attitudes and rules also play a part. As the old saying goes, nothing is certain in life but death and taxes, and both of these apply to estate planning. Let's first see how legal institutions influence an individual's or couple's decision to pass on wealth to their offspring. As Pestieau (2003) shows in his research on bequest motives, government regulations regarding wealth transmission are important influences on the financial and nonpecuniary behavior of parents and their desire for savings and consumption.

THE EFFECTS OF PUBLIC POLICY ON FAMILY GIFT GIVING

In the United States, legal institutions regulate welfare transfers in the form of two types of taxation: inheritance and estate taxes. Inheritance taxes are collected by states. Although the federal government does not levy an inheritance tax, it does impose an estate tax. Inheritance taxes are the oldest and most common form of "death tax." They are typically levied at graduated rates based on the amount of the bequest and on the relationship between the deceased and the beneficiary. Supporters of the inheritance tax see it as a way of ensuring that the wealthiest Americans pay a larger share of taxes or give away a larger share of their wealth to charity (Carasso and Steuerle, 2003). Detractors view it as a complex, unfair, and inefficient levy that penalizes the thriftiness of the deceased.

Since 1826, death taxes (i.e., inheritance and estate taxes) traditionally had been an area of state jurisdiction. Federal death taxes were levied intermittently from 1797 through 1915, but only to serve as a supplementary revenue source during wartime. In 1916, however, the federal government imposed a permanent estate tax. A controversy arose, as the states felt that the federal government was infringing on one of their traditional tax bases. The controversy heightened in the 1920s when state government finances became stressed. As the opposition increased, the federal government was forced to act.

In 1924, Congress offered a compromise. The federal estate tax rates were increased, but Congress provided for a credit of up to 25 percent against the federal tax for death taxes paid to the states. Under the Federal Estate Tax Act of 1926, the maximum credit increased from 25 percent to 80 percent. Today this credit is commonly referred to as a "pick-up" tax. As discussed earlier, the total tax liability for the beneficiaries does not increase and all states currently impose this tax up to the allowable federal credit.

The U.S. Tax Reform Act (TRA) of 1976 and the Economic Recovery Tax Act (ERTA) of 1981 brought about major changes in the administration of the pick-up tax, resulting in fewer estates being subject to the tax and sharply reduced taxes for those that were. This, in turn, resulted in less state revenue collected because state pick-up taxes are levied as a specified percentage of the federal estate tax. Most recently, federal estate tax law was changed by the 1997 Taxpayer Relief Act, which raised the $600,000 estate tax exemption ceiling to $700,000. In 2002, that amount was boosted to $1,000,000, under the Economic Growth and Tax Relief Reconciliation Act of 2001 (EGTRRA), and the limit will increase gradually to $2 million by 2008 and $3.5 million later in the decade (2009), again resulting in less state revenue collected under the pick-up tax. The historic act negated prior legislation designed to generate federal revenue by imposing a "death tax" on wealthier households.

Today, death taxes are imposed on transfers of property at the time of death or in anticipation of death when transfers are made two years before death.

HOW ESTATE TAXES VARY

Estate taxes are levied at graduated rates based on the value of the estate. Unlike the inheritance tax, the rates generally are imposed on the estate as a whole and do not vary based on the relationship of the beneficiary to the donor. However, there are exceptions. Although relief from estate taxes usually takes the form of a single specific exemption that applies to the entire estate, thereby reducing the taxable base, sometimes property transferred to specific kinds of beneficiaries, for example a surviving spouse, may be tax exempt. Oklahoma's law recognizes two separate classes: Lineal descendants are allowed a total aggregate deduction up to $175,000 while nonrelatives receive no deduction.

Estate tax rates vary a great deal across the country. In Ohio, for example, the rates range from 2 percent for taxable estates not exceeding $40,000 to 7 percent for taxable estates exceeding $500,000. In other states, like New York, estate taxes range from 2 percent for taxable estates up to $50,000 to 21 percent for taxable estates over $10 million.

The EGTRRA passed by a narrow vote of 51 to 48 in the Senate; it will be repealed at the end of 2010 and reinstated in 2011. The legislation is highly controversial and was hotly debated during the spring of 2001, for several reasons.

TABLE 7.1
Distribution of Estate Tax Liability (2000 Income Levels)

Income Category	Percentage of Income	Percentage of Estate and Gift Tax Liability
Bottom quintile	2.7	0.0
Second quintile	7.2	0.0
Third quintile	12.6	0.0
Fourth quintile	21.3	0.8
Top quintile	56.7	99.2
Top 10 percent	40.5	96.2
Top 5 percent	25.4	91.0
Top 1 percent	14.8	64.2

Source: Data from Burman and Gale, 2001; Cronin, 1999.
Note: The Treasury Department's tables are based on "family economic income," a broad-based income concept developed by the agency and used since the 1980s. The department has experimented with alternative income measures: the qualitative conclusions generally do not depend on the income measure.

Even some wealthy Americans opposed changes to the estate law. Most of the anger directed toward the reduction in tax schedule related to the widening income disparity observed between the rich and the poor (Gates and Collins, 2003). As Table 7.1 reveals, some policy makers have cause for concern because of the negative impact the reduction may have on charitable giving among wealthy households. The policy may create a situation in which there may be a reduction in the amount of charitable giving due to the smaller amount of money left in the estate at the time of death (Burman and Gale, 2001).

ESTATE TAXES AND EXEMPTIONS

The present inheritance tax law allows couples to exempt $2 million, as shown in Table 7.2. As earlier mentioned, by 2009, this exemption level will have risen to $3.5 million for an individual and $7 million for a couple. This amount is much higher for private businesses and family farm owners, who have long been given additional exemptions. Currently, with careful planning, businesses can pass on $5 million tax-free dollars. For farms, the amount equals $8 million. For the 2003 tax year, the average amount of the total estate taxes actually paid ranged between 45 and 49 percent. As Table 7.2 shows, however, after the $1 million basic exemption and other deductions are applied, the average effective estate tax rate—the percentage of the total estate actually paid in taxes—works out to be much lower. In 2001, the top rate was 60 percent; by 2005 this had dropped to 47 percent, and beginning in 2007 it drops to the bottom rate of 45 percent. In 2010, under current federal law, the estate tax will be eliminated entirely.

TABLE 7.2
Projections of Transfer Tax Exemptions and Rates Due to EGTRRA, 2001–2010

Calendar Year	Value of Estate and GST Tax Transfer Exemption	Highest Estate and Gift Tax Rates (%)
2001*	$ 675,000	60
2002	1,000,000	50
2003	1,000,000	49
2004	1,500,000	48
2005	1,500,000	47
2006	2,000,000	46
2007	2,000,000	45
2008	2,000,000	45
2009	3,500,000	45
2010	N/A (taxes repealed)	35 (gift tax only)

Source: Data from Burman and Gale, 2001.
*Pre-EGTRRA law.

Inheritance Tax

After the federal government levies taxes on the estate of the deceased person, states have the right to levy inheritance taxes on the person receiving the bequest. Five types of exemptions are usually allowed under inheritance tax laws: (1) personal exemptions based on the relationship of the giver and receiver; (2) exemptions of a specified amount allowed the entire estate; (3) exemptions for property on which a tax already has been paid; (4) exemptions for bequests to charitable, religious, or educational institutions; and (5) exemptions for particular types of property.

Of these five exemptions, the most significant is the personal exemption granted to beneficiaries based on their relationship to the decedent. Inheritance taxes are higher when property is left to distant relatives or friends; this encourages leaving estates to immediate family members. In South Dakota, for example, children's inheritance is taxed at rates varying from nothing on the first $30,000 to 7.5 percent for amounts exceeding $100,000. Surviving children also receive a $3,000 exemption. By contrast, nonrelatives are subject to rates ranging from 6 percent to 30 percent and receive only a $100 exemption.

Taxation rates vary tremendously from state to state. For example, in Indiana, lineal descendants are taxed at rates varying from 1 percent on inheritances of up to $25,000 to 10 percent on amounts of $1.5 million or more. In Pennsylvania, however, they are taxed at a 6 percent rate and nonrelatives are taxed at a 15 percent rate, regardless of the amount of inheritance. As Table 7.3 reveals, the results of variation in tax rates and credits creates large differences in the amount

TABLE 7.3
Estate Taxes, by State, 2000

State of Residence	Estates Taxed after Credits	
	Number	Amount
Alabama	530	246,696
Alaska	56*	7,537*
Arizona	858	340,702
Arkansas	229	103,028
California	8,365	3,677,278
Colorado	689	242,615
Connecticut	1,063	513,450
Delaware	261	151,899
District of Columbia	241	136,334
Florida	4,424	2,675,987
Georgia	668	520,768
Hawaii	357	128,000
Idaho	73	123,368
Illinois	2,702	1,182,176
Indiana	1,079	388,169
Iowa	572	173,832
Kansas	672	202,779
Kentucky	591	259,127
Louisiana	548	274,044
Maine	162	155,240
Maryland	1,001	405,231
Massachusetts	1,375	595,507
Michigan	1,527	680,959
Minnesota	672	220,420
Mississippi	231	82,172
Missouri	1,191	605,413
Montana	180	45,922
Nebraska	605	115,490
Nevada	118	187,551
New Hampshire	138	139,297
New Jersey	2,349	1,121,476
New Mexico	182	36,636
New York	3,963	2,379,134
North Carolina	1,025	460,897
North Dakota	80*	11,175*
Ohio	1,706	737,494
Oklahoma	709	143,385
Oregon	384	141,557
Pennsylvania	2,418	1,007,469
Rhode Island	177	107,780
South Carolina	400	148,545
South Dakota	111	57,752
Tennessee	662	297,737
Texas	2,577	1,119,884
Utah	191	231,336
Vermont	185	47,610
Virginia	1,268	538,220
Washington	1,133	398,983
West Virginia	250	97,770
Wisconsin	803	439,610
Wyoming	103	153,501
Total	52,000	24,398,622

Source: Data from Internal Revenue Service, 2006.
*Estimated quantities based on small sample of returns.

of inheritance taxes states collect. For estate tax reports filed in 2000, the total amount collected was more than $24 million, with California taking in the largest tax revenue and Alaska the smallest amount.

For most Americans, then, given the size of the estate subjected to statutory law, the government at any level plays a minor role in bequest motives. Only the most fortunate people pay federal estate taxes in the United States (Schervish and Havens, 2003). In fact, since the recent legal revisions, 98 percent do not. The wealthiest 2 percent of Americans are now the only ones who pay most of the estate taxes. Analyses of the 1998 General Social and Consumer Expenditures Surveys show that family households in the top 5 percent income tax bracket made up nearly 40 percent of philanthropic contributions (Schervish and Havens, 2003). In 2000, more than half of all estate taxes were paid by 3,621 people with estates larger than $5 million—representing the top 0.15 percent of all Americans. More than 2.4 million adults died in the United States in 2000, but only about 52,000 left taxable estates (Weisman, 2003). Thus, an extremely limited number of Americans are affected under the current legal regime. That said, it is critical for all individuals, no matter how prosperous, to be aware of legal factors affecting the tax threshold on which one can transfer wealth to heirs, however modest the amount.

Gift Tax

Closely related to death taxes are gift taxes. The gift tax is imposed on large transfers of wealth from living people. In general, any individual taxpayer can gift up to $12,000 to a family member or non–family member each year and there are no tax consequences. In fact, a person can make $11,000 gifts to as many different people in a year as she or he likes with no tax consequences. Spouses can give each other gifts of any amount without gift tax filings. Finally, a husband and wife can gift anyone $24,000 without gift tax consequences; but unless the husband gives $12,000 and the wife gives $12,000 and they each write a check, they will need to file a form with the IRS and elect to use gift splitting, which is when a husband and wife elect to treat a gift given by one of them as if half were given by each of them. In such a case, they will need to be careful about other gifts provided that year (e.g., birthdays, holidays) if they wish not to exceed the maximum amount.

ESTATE PLANNING FOR THE FAMILY

Elderly people, like everyone else, have a variety of legal problems, but some legal problems are found predominantly in the elderly population. Two intertwined problems facing elders are estate planning and managing one's assets to maintain a good standard of living in the later years. Most Americans are living much longer and much healthier lives. We also all have fewer children and less concentrated family structures. Consequently, we have to plan accordingly.

The family is the most important element in estate planning and in planning for one's later years (Cox, 2003). Estate planning is almost always precipitated by worries. Either the potential beneficiaries will encourage an elder to plan or the elder's concerns about his or her family will inspire planning. In many instances, families want to organize affairs so that the third generation will benefit; the elder's children don't see themselves as necessarily needing the wealth that the parent may pass down (Hendlin, 2004). But also, the more important planning that takes place, usually simultaneously with estate planning, is how one's wealth will be used to provide for one's long-term security in deep old age. That is almost always the most important issue to the child of an elderly person. Children generally are not the greedy, grasping people seen in soap operas or read about in the press. They generally are selfless and want their elderly parent to use the money and assets that they have accumulated to make themselves comfortable and safe in their later years. In the end, the greatest inheritance which any family can leave to its heirs must be a sense of security and making future generations successful.

Yet, the prospect of nursing home care can be stressful, and the decision-making process is complex, in large part because it may place a significant financial burden on an older parent and his or her family. Perhaps more importantly, estimates show that about 40 percent of people who turn 65 will use a nursing home at some point in their lives and many will need home care and other related services as well in the near future (Estes and Associates, 2001). According to the Health Insurance Association of America, by the year 2020, 12 million older Americans are expected to need long-term health care services. Seventy-five percent of elderly people in need of long-term care will be women in their midnineties as compared to 50 percent of men (Spillman and Lubitz, 2000).

Many elderly people consider themselves at low risk of financial impoverishment, believing that Medicare will pay for needed care if functional capacity is lost. Yet, paying for 24-hour-a-day long-term care in a nursing home can cost $40,000 to $80,000 per year. In 2005, a total of $207 billion was spent in private and public funds on long-term care in nursing homes and home health care services (Georgetown University Long-Term Care Financing Project, 2007).

In 2003, Medicaid paid for nearly half of the total cost of long-term care, approximately 47 percent, which went mostly to nursing facilities; followed by private out-of-pocket payments, 21 percent; Medicare, 18 percent; 9 percent private insurance; and 5 percent other public programs (O'Brien and Elias, 2004). Medicaid spending for long-term care services has tripled in the past twenty years, increasing from $21.1 billion in 1987 to $56.1 billion in 1997 and then climbing to $95 billion in 2005.

In 2006, the average cost of a nursing home stay was $194 per day for a private room, but the costs of long-term care vary widely, running twice as high in some regions of the nation than in others (MetLife [Mature Market Institute Survey], 2002). In Alaska, for example, the average nursing home rate is $524 per day (U.S. Department of Health and Human Services, 2007). The comptroller general of the United States predicts that this trend will continue for decades to come (General Accounting Office, 2002).

Two-thirds of nursing home residents now rely on Medicaid to pay for their care. Between 14 and 35 percent of those admitted to nursing homes as private-pay residents spend down their funds until they become eligible for Medicaid. This is because Medicare does not cover long-term nursing home care for people who are not financially needy. Nor will the program pay for intermediate-level care, provided at assisted living facilities, for elderly people who need only limited assistance with activities of daily living, such as meal preparation, medication, and transportation. This fact leaves a serious gap in the overall safety net for elderly people. Medicaid, intended to be the health care financing option of last resort, has become the payer for the majority of nursing home residents.

What families often do not realize, though, is that most middle-class families do not qualify for Medicaid benefits, because it is a means-tested program with strict guidelines for financial eligibility (Stum, 1998). To qualify for Medicaid nursing home benefits, a recipient must: (1) be admitted to an approved Medicaid nursing home under a physician's orders; (2) have medical and nursing care expenses that exceed income; and (3) have only $2,000 or less of nonexempt assets, excluding a home for a nonmarried applicant or $66,000 in such assets and their home for a married couple. Among those who enter nursing homes as private-pay residents, nearly 70 percent reach the poverty level after three months; 90 percent within one year. The Omnibus Budget Reconciliation Act of 1993 (OBRA 1993) (referred to as the Deficit Reduction Act) extended the "look back period," the period for which one is ineligible for Medicaid due to disqualifying transfers: before OBRA '93, there was an upper limit on ineligibility of 30 months; under OBRA '93 there is no upper limit or 60 months for trusts (Sevak and Walker, 2007).

Although Medicaid rules require beneficiaries to use up most of their assets in nursing facility payments before Medicaid begins, there are ways to preserve many of those assets. Each option has some drawbacks, however, and not all of them will be available for everyone. Different methods pertain to unmarried people and to couples; some require advanced planning and the assistance of a lawyer or other professional advisor. A trust can be used to preserve some assets for future generations. Current regulations involving trusts are complex; in some circumstances they require that the assets of the trust be used to repay Medicaid after the death of the Medicaid recipient. But in most cases, strategic care planning can help an elderly person and his or her family reduce the burden of nursing home costs. In addition, the individual can keep assets of certain trusts that include the Medicaid recipient as a beneficiary. With that said, critics note that the current system creates perverse incentives for middle-class elderly people—that they "spend down" to meet the poverty threshold for Medicaid long-term care benefits by sheltering or divesting themselves of their financial assets (Burwell and Crown, 1994).

PRIVATE LONG-TERM CARE INSURANCE

Long-term care insurance is an insurance contract that, in exchange for a premium, covers some or all expenses when full-time nursing assistance is needed, whether in a nursing facility, in a community-based setting, or at home, after a predetermined waiting period, called an "elimination period." Long-term care insurance does not cover acute care in a hospital. Estimates vary on the proportion of consumers able to afford private long-term care insurance, and they range from as low as 6 percent to as high as 40 percent. About 1.5 million Americans own a private long-term care insurance policy (Angel, 2001). For a growing number of aging Baby Boomers, this is a legitimate way of staying in control of their assets while also maximizing choice in long-term care options.

Because so few people own policies, Congress elevated the issue at the dawn of the twenty-first century. The importance of making long-term care insurance affordable and accessible was underscored by the federal Long-term Care Security Act signed into law on September 19, 2000 (U.S. Office of Personnel Management, 2006). The law provides private long-term care insurance for more than 13 million federal employees and their families. The plan covers personal care, home health care, adult day care, and nursing home care at premiums that are 15 to 20 percent lower than the cost of private plans. As a result of this legislation and aggressive marketing efforts, a total of 5.8 million people had long-term care insurance policies in 2001.

ESTATE RECOVERY AND RELATED LONG-TERM CARE
FINANCING ISSUES

As part of Omnibus Budget Reconciliation Act of 1993, the rules for Medicaid eligibility determination were significantly changed (U.S. Department of Health and Human Services, 2005). The federal government ordered the states to begin seeking reimbursement for long-term care costs from Medicaid recipients' estates. These changes were designed to discourage Medicaid estate planning, the process whereby a person divests or transfers assets to others in order to become eligible for Medicaid. This practice is primarily used to avoid spending one's own wealth to pay for long-term care by having Medicaid pay for it. This tactic is often referred to as "gaming" and has significant implications for bequests.

More than half of the states enacted some estate recovery legislation between 1982 and 1993, although not all of the states enacted legislation to implement programs to recover Medicaid recipients' estates. The cost effectiveness of estate recovery varies from state to state. According to the General Accounting Office (GAO), Oregon spent $306,000 to recover $4,000,000 but Rhode Island spent $26,000 to recover only $45,000 in 1989 (General Accounting Office, 1989).

In 1993, the top ten estate-recovery programs managed to collect about 1 percent of the total cost of nursing home care. The total amount states collected was $124.8 million in 1995, less than one-half of 1 percent of that year's nursing home expenditures. There are several reasons for variations in estate recovery. First, probate law is the domain of the states and varies dramatically among them. Some states give Medicaid a higher priority claim on an estate's funds than others do. In Texas, for example, the Medicaid claim is a sixth-class claim, following funeral expenses, last illness expenses, expenses of administration of the estate, secured claims (e.g., a mortgage or car loan), taxes, and claims by the Texas Department of Criminal Justice for the costs of confinement (Texas Probate Code #322). A second factor is related to the amount of the Medicaid recipient's estate, namely, family allowance and personal property set aside for surviving spouse and/or dependent child. In Texas, the personal property set-aside can protect as much as $60,000 in some instances and the family allowance is at the court's discretion. And, third, how much of the estate passes through probate is another factor influencing the amount states recover. Probate may be avoided through the use of trusts and property that passes to the co-owner at the Medicaid recipient's death.

INTER VIVOS TRANSFERS AND INHERITANCE

When should one begin the process of estate planning and when should the family members get involved? What is the decision-making process underlying gifting either by inter vivos or by bequest? The dynamic of gift giving has piqued the interest of those outside government because of the expected wealth transfers to heirs and to other individuals and organizations in decades to come. As Chapter 1 stated, the amount is projected to be at least $41 trillion (Havens and Schervish, 1999). But families, financial advisors, and attorneys are often at a loss as to how to make these financial decisions (Schervish and Havens, 2003).

Research by attorneys indicates that the first stage of estate planning should begin as soon as one needs to provide for a spouse, partner, or other dependent (Farrell, 2001). Most people start thinking about passing along assets when they have children. However, the literature suggests that many elders are afraid to do end-of-life planning for themselves or their spouse (Pestieau, 2003). Confronting death and illness is an act fraught with foreboding. But once people get past the fear, they tend to realize that what they consider to be selfless giving to others actually just shifts the burden of caring for themselves to the next generation. An elder's loved ones will have to do whatever it takes to care for him or her (Angel and Angel, 1997).

It is important to recognize that an inter vivos gift is a transfer of the donor's assets to the recipient, usually a child or a spouse, so the recipient has these assets to take care of him- or herself, not the donor. Contributions to college education and paying for medical care for someone who is ill are both examples of inter vivos transfers. These transfers involve taking one's property and gifting it to another, including grandchildren. In the process, those assets cease to be a part of one's estate. They may or may not be available to help in a later situation of need.

While it may seem that these transfer tools—gifts and bequests—are simple and apply to everyone equally, serious problems may arise when an older person makes such transfers but does not develop a long-range plan. No two families are exactly alike when it comes to giving, and a great deal of damage is often done by improperly making inter vivos transfers. Such actions are sometimes based on insufficiently grounded motivation, like what the next-door neighbors learned from their lawyer or watching a friend struggle with a financial problem. Frequently, it is that rumor or gossip that makes someone want to start giving away their property "so that the government will not get it." This is a common misperception among elderly people. The best way to be informed about one's personal financial situation is to take stock of current and future income and assets and to analyze them with family members, legal counsel, or with a financial planner (Schervish and Havens, 2003). This is especially true when making decisions about financing long-term care (Angel, 1999) and making bequests to philanthropic organizations (Schervish and Havens, 2003).

THE IMPACT OF GIFT GIVING ON THE FAMILY: WHAT HELPS? WHAT HURTS?

Contributions to college education, perhaps medical expenses for adult children, and even, in some cases, grandchildren, may affect the estate and the amount of the estate in the future. Research shows that, even among the most wealthy Americans, individuals and couple-headed households are not aware of how to build a secure nest egg (Kennickell, Starr-McCluer, and Sundén, 1996). Some older adults are completely at a loss when trying to gauge their future financial situation. The greatest concern centers on how to weigh savings relative to spending, or gifting, as one grows older (Bernheim, Schleifer, and Summers, 1985). For Baby Boomers, the high costs of education are fueling many of these emotions. Should tuition costs be factored into inheritance? Should your children have to wait until you are dead to receive all of their inheritance?

Survey data suggest that many elderly persons have a fairly rudimentary knowledge of financial planning and that often intentions are not correlated with expected, or precautionary, savings behavior (Bernheim et al., 1985). Gustman and Steinmeier (2003) provide empirical evidence showing that few elderly Americans are aware of their Social Security and Medicare benefits. Likewise, the conventional wisdom is that graying Baby Boomers approaching their retirement years are not effectively planning how to allocate their income between spending and saving (Hurd and Smith, 2002).

The American Bar Association Section of Real Property, Probate and Trust Law recommends keeping a notebook that includes everything important about a person's assets and all of their estate planning documents, such as powers of attorney (American Bar Association, 2002). One of the most important things to have in a notebook is a copy of the signature card of every bank account one holds and every financial brokerage account. This is crucial because a lot of inadvertent estate planning gets done at the bank. Ironically, much of estate planning is not integrated with services provided by an attorney or financial planner or accountant. Preparing this notebook enables another family member to make decisions if an elder is temporarily or permanently incapacitated and cannot make decisions.

Such a notebook is one of the most loving things one can do for one's family, and should be provided to any person with a durable power of attorney. And it greatly facilitates the use of the services of a lawyer or a financial planner or an accountant. The professional can actually help make the process efficient, because he or she can see the whole picture of how the assets are working for the client and for his or her spouse and children.

Making good decisions about who will have legal access to one's assets is fraught with difficulties, however. For instance, there are dangers in accounts that are established with joint tenancy with right of survivorship. This type of arrangement could take all the assets within that account out of an individual's estate. How could this happen? If you open an account with someone else on that account for convenience's sake, that person is a cosigner, along with you, on that account. That cosigner can sign checks drawn on that account. Upon your death, that joint-tenant account becomes the property of the cosigner, by right of survivorship. If you bequeathed what is in that account to someone other than that cosigner, the beneficiary may have no legal access to that account. That simple illustration shows how a great deal of well-intended estate planning can be undone. But such troubles can be minimized by having joint tenancy on only an account with a small amount of money used for day-to-day expenses.

Many times conflicts arise because of the mismanagement of banking and brokerage accounts. This is also true of individual retirement accounts (IRAs), for which assigning a beneficiary is an important component of the planning. However, the failure to set up and integrate those accounts with one's will and estate plan can cause a great deal of the assets that have been acquired to be distributed in a manner contrary to one's wishes.

Every family has its own ideology, and often it is difficult for elder parents to communicate with the adult children about their needs, about their concerns, including who will be the executor of the will, because discussing money is uncomfortable for most families. It is clear from the research that elderly parents express their gift-giving intentions in a variety of ways but that decisions about gifts naturally must work within the confines of the law and their financial situation. These decisions may depend on social class, ethnicity, religion, and other factors related to the timing of life-course transitions, such as divorce. Some parents clearly see money as one means of cementing the bonds with their children. Others separate the meaning of money from emotional ties and do not give gifts to their adult children. Generally, most families see leaving and receiving inheritances as an act of love from one generation to the next.

From a practical point of view, ensuring that these people's wishes come to fruition can be impeded by problems, often as a result of family feuds, despite the donor's well-meaning intentions. So what can be done to ensure that preferences about one's personal financial legacy are realized? Below I discuss the array of practical issues related to intergenerational wealth transfers facing aging families today.

Ideally, if one has assets that exceed basic living needs, then it will be worth spending the hour or so with a lawyer, or at least with an accountant, that is necessary to discuss the writing of a will. Also, if one has any savings, life insurance, or real property, seeking professional help can alleviate a lot of unnecessary heartache after you are gone.

MYTHS AND REALITIES OF MAKING A WILL

A will is a legal document of instructions on what should happen to one's assets when one dies. The will can also include burial instructions. If one spouse dies without a will, state law might force the other spouse to split the assets of the estate with the children, leaving the surviving spouse without enough support. Stepchildren, ex-spouses still living, noncustodial children, and a myriad of other possible heirs can add further complications. When preparing a will without the assistance of an attorney, it is important to study one's state probate statutes to find out precisely what the law requires for a will to be considered acceptable in court. Who needs a will? Ideally, if you have assets that exceed basic living expenses you should make some sort of will.

Structuring how assets are to be directed toward the care of the person who accumulated them as old age sets in may involve considering catastrophic health care spending. Care planning must include arrangements should the person become mentally incapacitated. Powers of attorney and wills need to be prepared and signed before a person becomes mentally incapacitated.

Sometimes, if a person becomes mentally incapacitated and is unable to make an actual will, he or she can still understand enough to, with help, prepare a living will or advanced medical directive. This document directs physicians, on paper, what to do in the event that the person becomes terminally ill and there is no hope for recovery (Prendergast, 2001). The advanced directive may include the name of a person who will make decisions about life-sustaining medical care, if more flexibility is desired than the decision written down (Angel, 1999). A medical power of attorney, which is another form of advanced directive recognized by most states, allows an individual to appoint someone to act on his or her behalf about any and all health care decisions (Stoeckle, Doorley, and McArdle, 1998). It can ensure that your life will not be prolonged, and your assets drained, if it is not your desire to be kept alive under certain circumstances.

Another tool that is useful if one thinks that it is possible one may become incapacitated is called a living trust. This is a trust into which one's assets can all be transferred. In this situation a child, a trusted advisor, or a banker has trust capacity and can operate that trust for the benefit of the elderly person when his or her capacity is gone. On the person's death, the assets are already owned by the trust and there is no probate of those assets. They just pass in whatever way the wording of the trust directs.

State law provides, as it does in every other situation, a default set of rules that apply if one fails to assign someone to act as agent of one's affairs in the event of functional incapacity. The law will, at the worst-case scenario, allow someone to apply to become the person's guardian. If this occurs, it is a failure of planning. Usually, when a guardian has to be appointed, the person who is now incapacitated has neglected to plan for that possibility. Sometimes, more rarely, the situation is the product of meddling by people who are self-interested in the plan, and others involved in the care of the client must come to the person's aid.

A will is not valid until the date of the person's death and then only after it is probated. A will can be changed by the writer up until the moment of death. There is even a provision in the law for death bed wills. Death bed wills are not planning devices, however. Few people on their death beds have the presence of mind to worry about anything other than their own illness. How their assets will be distributed after their death is a secondary consideration.

In the end, the most important thing adult children can do is to set aside their own interests and listen to the parents. They should ask the hard questions: "Dad, you know you're not going to live forever; you may become ill at some point. Tell us what you want us to do. Give us our marching orders." Don't worry about whether there's going to be anything left. Take mom and dad to a competent lawyer and make sure their preferences are set down in writing in a way that will pass legal muster and will actually be carried out.

Even if there are no pressing health care concerns, there are some social situations that can change the terms of a will. Situations that existed at the time of the original will's preparation are subject to change. All of the following are circumstances that might prompt someone to change his or her will: (1) having provided for a child who has since died, (2) providing for grandchildren who now have become quite capable of taking care of themselves, (3) having remarried, and (4) having children by a prior marriage who may expect inheritance but preferring to provide for one's current spouse. Also, many people make the mistake of angering family members by making on paper a plan that does not match what they have told their family they are going to do. That comes, again, out of that caring desire not to damage or hurt a family relationship, perhaps with one's child or one's spouse. Of course, ongoing communication with family is crucial in the operative planning and creation and maintenance of a will.

As discussed, many factors influence how parents distribute their assets, and changes in an heir's circumstances may cause changes in a will. Most parents expect to be equal with the distribution of their estates, in part, because they do not want to show favoritism or cause any resentment. However, equal treatment can be difficult when one child has done well and another is struggling in life. The ability to give to a child, especially to one who has financial woes, is also a reflection of a parent's own success. Individual parents will vary in how they handle such situations.

Sibling Rivalry

What can happen to gift and inheritances processes when siblings don't get along and conflicts arise? Conflicts between sisters and brothers are inevitable. A parent whose children are prone to argue should go to a lawyer when creating his or her will, because there are efficient processes under state law that can help avoid sibling fights, help resolve them, or put assets beyond the reach of the sibling fight; although the fight may continue to rage, it will not damage one's estate plan.

However, if estate planning does not occur and the state courts step in to distribute assets, a great deal of the estate's money may need to be spent for lawyers, legal processes, and hearings. When the probate process is completed, such estates are often depleted, so it pays to make your wishes known in writing.

If you can foresee that there will be conflict of interest between children and a current spouse or partner, and a parent has definite wishes about how assets should be divided, it is important to understand the steps you should take. For example, if one wants a new spouse to provide care for oneself but any remaining money to go to one's children or grandchildren, drawing up a prenuptial or post-nuptial agreement stating how those assets will be characterized and distributed across interested parties is useful. The best way to avoid conflict among children if you have remarried is to combine your planning with that of your spouse while you are still alive.

An Accountant or Elder Attorney?

Good estate planning usually requires more than one type of professional—there isn't really a one-stop shop for estate planning. Many people rely solely on their accountants for financial planning and will simply tack on estate planning. Such an accountant would need to know as much as possible about asset accumulation. It is important to explore whether you can avoid estate taxes and to determine if your assets are set up to efficiently pass to the designated beneficiaries. Accountants and financial planners are a good first stop, but there is important knowledge that an elder law attorney can bring to the planning process. A lawyer, on the other hand, is a poor substitute for a financial planner. The work that the accountant and the financial planner do not only helps provide for your current needs, such as income tax or investment counseling, but also helps you focus all of your attention on the broader asset picture. Once that view is complete, a lawyer can then efficiently help you plan how your assets will be distributed.

Long-Term Care

Spending down assets or sheltering assets to ensure a legacy may result in a serious decline in capacity to pay for a long illness. Medicare does not cover the costs of long-term care, in a nursing home or in the community. For this reason, buying private long-term care insurance may increase the likelihood that assets will be passed on to one's heirs. Research shows that the need for long-term care will be growing in years to come (Angel and Angel, 1997). As Chapter 1 illustrated, covering the costs of that care will increasingly be burdensome for the vast majority of elderly Americans, because of the price of nursing home care. The price of long-term care insurance premiums is out of the financial reach of many low- and moderate-income elderly persons. In addition, Americans are now having fewer children, and adult children from all social groups are less able than in the past to take care of their elderly parents (Angel and Angel, 1997).

The desire to leave an inheritance is frequently the reason an older person is willing to consider purchasing long-term care insurance. Clearly, the issue of covering costs for long-term care affects estate planning, but it also affects the ultimate well-being of families. One of the reasons for estate planning among wealth holders is to avoid spending capital assets (Schervish and Havens, 2003). For those individuals who have sufficient assets and income to provide for the "worst-case scenario," long-term care insurance is a concrete method of increasing the likelihood of leaving a legacy for someone else. Buying private long-term care insurance can protect a certain amount of *income* for those who want to leave more of the money which would go to payments for nursing home care or home health services. A long-term care insurance policy allows the client to predict with more assurance that an inheritance of at least a certain value will be available.

As the Baby Boom Generation ages, many more people will need to plan for retirement and save for it, because future corporate pension systems may not be able to honor obligations promised to employees (Walsh, 2005) and many employers are no longer making such promises. In Chapter 8, I take a look at the social and economic policies designed to address the problems and challenges of supporting the welfare of children and aged people.

CHAPTER EIGHT

Inheritance and the Next Generation of Old-Age Policies

Where, where but here have pride and truth
That long to give themselves for wage,
To shake their wicked sides at youth
Restraining reckless middle-age?
—W. B. Yeats (1865–1939)

The major challenges facing benefactors are family communication and governmental taxing policies. Most families see leaving and receiving inheritances as an act of love between generations. The taxing authorities see estate taxes as a way to increase their coffers.

The state has another vested interest in beneficial inheritance practices, because of the economic impact they have on younger workers and future generations. The government needs for as much wealth as possible to be passed on to the next generation. Why? As some critics, such as Alan Greenspan, former chairman of the Federal Reserve Board, argue, in the near future, entitlement programs will no longer be available to retirees, and consequently, senior citizens will bear a larger responsibility to provide for their own well-being. The payroll taxes that they paid all their working career have not gone toward their own retirement but support the current class of retirees. When Generations X and Y get ready to retire, there will not be enough workers contributing to payroll taxes to support them, and the majority of workers who are left will be poor minorities. These retirees will be ostensibly on their own. Hence, well-managed estates, no matter how modest, will play an important role in the financial safety net of future retirees. The historic social programs put into place for retirees, namely Social Security and Medicare, will be history (Kingson and Reinhardt, 2000).

Others commentators vociferously disagree, however. Many sociologists and antiprivatization economists label these statements as hyperbole, believing that there is no actuarial basis for making these claims. They contend that these estimates are based on conservative assumptions. They concede that the "crisis" rhetoric has created a fear among young workers that the program will not be there when they reach retirement age. These analysts have a different opinion about the outlook of the old-age assistance programs. They dismiss the dismal forecast that the Social Security Trust Fund will "go broke" for pure methodological reasons, because, in their scenario, the U.S. economy will grow at a rate of 2.4 percent between now and 2042. But the U.S. economy has grown 3–4 percent over the past 80 years—and that includes the Great Depression of the 1930s. All we need is economic growth of 2.8 percent and there will be no decrease in benefits for Generations X and Y.

Baker and Weisbrot (1999) concur with the second interpretation. They believe that, under current projections in the 2005 Social Security Trustees Report, the Social Security Federal Old-Age and Survivors Insurance Program (OASI) can honor benefits to retirees as promised for the next forty years. Another reason they believe this is feasible is that the relative amount of payroll taxes is far less than what has been observed in previous decades, about 1.89 percent. The researchers recommend that policy makers consider raising the cap on income subject to Social Security tax, which in 2005 was the first $90,000 of wages. Some moderate Republican lawmakers, such as Olympia Snowe, also voice concern over the notion that Social Security is in crisis and that the system should be overhauled. She does not want to support President Bush's proposal to divert a portion of the Federal Insurance Contribution Act payroll taxes to private accounts, testifying in front of the Senate Finance Committee that it would exacerbate the anticipated benefits shortage (Neikirk, 2005).

THE NEW STATUS QUO

Old-age security is becoming an important issue worldwide. Chapter 3 underlined the generous support systems for older individuals that were put in place during times of rapid economic growth and which are now an integral part of the political economies of developed nations. To bring home this point once again,

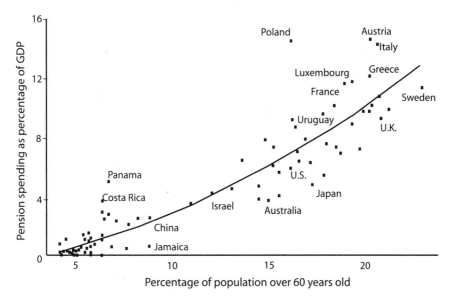

Figure 8.1. Relationship between Percentage of the Population over 60 Years Old and Public Pension Spending. *Source:* Data from World Bank, 1994.

Figure 8.1 shows that many industrialized countries now spend more than 10 percent of their GDP on pensions (Dang, Antolin, and Oxley, 2001). In some industrialized nations, public spending on health and pensions now exceeds 20 percent of the gross domestic product (James, 2001). Spending for old-age pensions is projected to consume another three to four percentage points of the GDP in most industrialized countries by the year 2050 (Dang et al., 2001). Unfortunately, with the arrival of the twenty-first century, the rapid economic growth that accompanied industrialization has slowed, and social welfare states face serious conflicts related to the cost of human services (Holzmann and Stiglitz, 2001).

What are the various scenarios for the future welfare of aging families based on potential changes in the world economy? If real economic growth in the United States and other developed countries remains relatively flat in years to come, some public officials argue, increased expenditures for elderly people can come only at the expense of other social goods, such as programs for children (Lamm, 2003). Even when aggregate wealth is high, slow growth will result in heated debates and conflicts over how our aggregate economic pie is to be divided (Kingson and Berkowitz, 1994).

Since the advent of Social Security, children no longer expect to be financially responsible for their aging parents (Crystal, 1984). Such a responsibility would be increasingly difficult, because life expectancies are longer and middle-aged individuals frequently find themselves responsible for both dependent children and aging parents. In the coming century, the pact between the generations will inevitably change (Munnell, 2003). Even now, the older generation is consuming resources at a rate that will leave those that come after them unable to pay the bill.

The notion that children must support their aging parents served well when most individuals died earlier than they do today and when their needs in old age were limited. If elderly people consume the lion's share of the aggregate production of society, we must wonder what the consequences of a geriatric society will be. In this chapter, I look at the expectations of middle-class Americans to maintain their lifestyle in retirement and consider the potential consequences of different levels of governmental support for elderly people. In that context, I examine the potential racial and ethnic tensions that may result from the fact that a larger proportion of the workforce will consist of blacks and Hispanics, while the older retired population will continue to be predominantly non-Hispanic white and politically and economically powerful.

SORTING OUT THE DEBATE

At the macro social level, it is clear that inequalities in income and wealth exist between the young and the old. Historically, the old have received more from the welfare state than the young (Angel and Angel, 1993). Spending on Social Security retirement and health insurance has far outpaced spending on programs for children needing public assistance, as shown in Table 8.1. In fiscal year 2000, the federal government spent a little over one-third of its budget—about $615 billion —on transfer payments and services for people age 65 and older (Congressional Budget Office, 2000). Federal spending, including entitlement and discretionary programs, on children in 2000 totaled about $148 billion. Entitlement programs accounted for the overwhelming share of the spending on elderly people (97 percent) but a much smaller portion of spending on families with children (about 67 percent). Over the next 10 years, under current policies, spending on elderly people and children combined will account for more than one-half of total government spending, with the elderly population making up 80 percent of that amount.

Not including effects of inflation, federal spending on the average retiree is estimated to rise from nearly $17,700 in 2000 to more than $21,100 in 2010. By contrast, federal spending on children will increase only from $2,100 in 2000 to about $2,500 by 2010. How our society perceives the difference in governmental

TABLE 8.1
Estimated Federal Spending for Elderly People under Selected Programs,
Fiscal Years 1980–2010

	1980	1990	2000	2010
Total federal spending on people 65 or over (billions of dollars)	$144	$360	$615	$1,050
Percentage of the budget	24.3%	28.7%	34.8%	42.8%
Percentage of gross domestic product	5.3%	6.3%	6.4%	7.1%
Per elderly person (in 2000 dollars)	$11,839	$15,192	$17,688	$21,122

Source: Data from Congressional Budget Office, 2000.

expenditures on the support of the elderly versus that of the very young is poorly understood.

Curiously, Americans of all age groups have not focused on generational equity. Consistent with evidence reported in the 1970s and 1980s, a recent AARP study found that little intergenerational conflict was reported by adults aged 18 and over. Granted, the survey results indicated that older Americans were not getting more than their fair share of local government resources; yet, younger adults believed that older people generally tend to oppose paying for services that do not benefit themselves, like property tax increases for local school improvements (Speas and Obenshain, 1995). Whether or not any of these attitudes vary across groups from different economic backgrounds is unknown.

What we do know is that those of us who will be retired will look to the young for support, in one form or another. If they are unable to provide it, our retirement years could be bleak. In a survey of adults' attitudes toward intergenerational relations in American society, more than 40 percent of respondents 35 and older without any savings believed that their retirement security was at risk. Although the vast majority of people have already begun saving for retirement, those of low or moderate means are finding saving for retirement difficult. They believe it will become a serious problem in their ability to pass on material gifts and wealth to their children (Princeton Survey Research Associates, 1998). This is significant, because members of future generations believe that their pathway to financial security will not depend on Social Security retirement benefits (Princeton Survey Research Associates, 1998). Instead, security will be achieved from their own savings and whatever inheritances they receive.

The contract binding generations is changing. At least four major issues are regularly discussed within the context of generational equity: the allocation of resources between older adults and their children, the concern over large governmental deficits, the distribution of health care resources to groups with competing claims, and the fairness of financing of Social Security by younger generations.

Some influential factors are either entirely absent from the discussion or are given only obligatory recognition when mentioned: class, race, ethics, and historical perspectives. In the following discussion, I posit ways in which this debate could shift from generational dependence to generational interdependence.

Toward that end, I include examples that exemplify the role of intergenerational transfers, including family caregiving and support of dependent elders across all segments of the population, especially as they affect the poor, many of whom are members of historically underrepresented minority groups, such as African Americans and Hispanics of Mexican origin. It is unclear the extent to which government support of retired persons will alter the behavior between older adults and their adult children and grandchildren. As Chapter 2 showed, population aging will influence the obligations and expectations across age groups, owing to dramatic demographic trends. Minority Americans represent not only the absolute increase in the number of individuals over 65 that poses problems but also the increase in the proportion of the total population (Angel and Angel, 2006). Judging by post–World War II fertility patterns, the proportion of persons over 65 will increase in all developed nations well into the next century. An increase in the ratio of older to younger individuals means that there are fewer employed individuals to support each retired person, resulting in a disproportionate flow of resources from the young to the old (Kingson and Reinhardt, 2000). Other research is less pessimistic, however, noting that the workers-to-retirees ratio ignores another factor of American life, namely higher levels of productivity with each passing year. Two workers produced in 2005 what it took nine workers to do in 1940. Technological innovation, for instance telecommunications and word processing, has vastly increased worker output (Galbraith and Berner, 2001).

But, is not the real problem the growing disparity between the rich and poor, not the one between the young and old? Hard evidence indicates that the potential dependency burden of the elderly population will fall especially on lower- and middle-class working families. That problem alone may give rise to new political and fiscal crises of the welfare state. Differences in the racial and ethnic composition of various age categories that result from differences in fertility and from immigration patterns have serious implications for resource flows and political conflict between the generations (Williamson, Watts-Roy, and Kingson, 1999).

POSSIBLE SCENARIOS

Just consider a country in which one-fifth of the population is retired and most of those retirees are white non-Latinos who have come to expect cost of living increases in Social Security and adequate Medicare coverage. Imagine that in this country the working population that supports these retirees is made up primarily of Latinos and other historically underrepresented minority groups. Imagine further that many of those workers (but not all who can successfully incorporate into society) are stuck in low-paying jobs because they face structural barriers that prevent adequate education and training to obtain good jobs that a high-tech, information-based economy creates and demands.

In this imaginary country, these young workers struggle to educate their children, to pay off mortgages, to provide health insurance for their families, and to save for their own retirement on small paychecks. Many find those paychecks shrunk by up to 40 percent by the Social Security and Medicare taxes that are required to support the older group (Palmer and Saving, 2004). Will these workers bear this burden without protest? Will the strain, made worse by ethnic and racial differences, add to resentment and conflict between the generations?

Such a scenario sounds sensationalistic, but it illustrates what problems we could face in our increasingly ethnically and economically diverse nation. Unfortunately, poverty, low education and family disruption continue to plague minority populations, making many young Latinos and African Americans poorly prepared to succeed in the economy of the twenty-first century. Simple demographics, however, mean that they will make up an ever-larger fraction of the working age population.

At the dawn of the twenty-first century, the U.S. population is aging rapidly, and the pact across the generations is both as simple as it has always been and yet far more complex. In conjunction with advances in the technical management of chronic disease, during what is likely to be a period of slow economic growth, this fact will lead to an increase in the political and economic strains associated with the care of the frail and disabled elderly population. A complicating factor in this scenario is the increasing cultural heterogeneity among elderly Americans. For example, elderly minorities will grow two to three times faster than the older population as a whole; they increased by 16 percent in 2000. By the year 2030, the projected number of elderly Latinos, African Americans, and other races is expected to reach almost 19 million. In the future, an ever-larger fraction of the older population will consist of individuals whose long-term medical care needs—and preferences in living arrangements—may differ significantly from those of the majority.

Even now, the United States looks much different than it did a decade ago. The stunning increase in the minority elderly population projected for the middle of this century will include, in addition to the 14 million Hispanics, 8.6 million blacks and 5.8 million persons of other non-white races. Although these numbers are truly remarkable, the reality could be even more dramatic if life expectancy among minorities improves more sharply than current projections assume (Elo and Preston, 1997). These compositional shifts have important implications for public policy dealing with social welfare, housing, and medical care.

Demographers also note that Hispanics—comprised of Mexicans (61%), Central and South Americans (11%), Puerto Ricans (12%), Cubans (5%), and all others (11%)—are one of the fastest growing segments of the U.S. population (Tienda and Mitchell, 2006). Almost three-quarters of the nation's Hispanics resided in California, Texas, New York, Florida, or Illinois in 2003 (U.S. Census Bureau, 2004b). The Hispanic population is growing almost five times faster than the general population. Since July 1, 1990, the Hispanic population has grown 29 percent, while the non-Hispanic white population has increased just 3 percent. Because of high fertility and immigration rates, the Hispanic population surpassed African Americans as the largest U.S. minority ethnic group in 2001 (U.S. Census Bureau, 2003). By the middle of this century, it is estimated, one of every four Americans will be Hispanic. What makes this population unique is that the average Hispanic American is much younger than the average non-Hispanic; about half of Hispanic Americans were under 26.5 years of age in 1998. Roughly one out of every three Hispanic Americans is under the age of 18 (Angel and Angel, 2006).

Currently, 80 percent of Hispanic men 16 years and over are in the labor force, the highest participation rate of any group. As a result of a young age structure combined with a swiftly rising population, middle-aged Hispanics are experiencing a midlife cycle squeeze that results from the simultaneous responsibility for children and aging parents. Although the majority of Hispanic households are married-couple families (55.5%), almost 20 percent are headed by women. Under these family circumstances, intergenerational exchanges of any sort are further strained as single mothers struggle to make ends meet.

More than likely, the sheer size of the population over 65 will make reductions in Social Security and Medicare inevitable. Individuals will simply have to pay higher taxes on their retirement earnings and pay a larger share of the Medicare they receive. One of the more disturbing possibilities that could result is increasing inequality between the rich and the poor among those over 65.

It is expected that, as at other times in history, this income inequality will closely follow racial and ethnic lines, generating even greater potential for divisions in our society. As Chapter 2 discussed, members of the Baby Boom Generation will be the beneficiaries of the greatest transfer of wealth in history as they inherit the assets of their parents. Experts expect that from 1998 through 2018, the parents of Baby Boomers and some aging Boomers themselves will leave estates worth more than $12 trillion to $18 trillion, the largest generational transfer of wealth in history. Although that enormous wealth transfer will include as many as 2.8 million estates worth $1 million or more over the next twenty years, many black and Hispanic heirs will not be the beneficiaries of these assets, owing to the accumulated economic disadvantages associated with minority group member-ship (Havens and Schervish, 1999).

THE POLITICS OF SOCIAL SECURITY REFORM

It is hardly surprising that both liberal and conservative politicians are avoiding the topic of Social Security reform. A few years ago, the Congressional Budget Office (CBO) reported that Social Security had enough taxes and interest owed to it from the U.S. Treasury to pay full benefits indefinitely.

But that was then; this is now. The trustees for Medicare and Social Security are taking a long-term budgetary outlook, and the picture they are painting is not very pretty. The board of trustees of the Social Security Trust Fund is composed of the secretary of the treasury, the secretary of labor, the secretary of health and human services, the commissioner of social security, and two members appointed by the president and confirmed by the Senate to serve as public representatives. The board publishes an annual report that forecasts the solvency of the Medicare and Social Security retirement programs. The trustees are projecting that both programs will be unable to meet their future benefit obligations (Palmer and Saving, 2004). This is mainly because of large looming shortfalls in funding the next generation of benefits. Some Democrats fault President Bush's tax cuts. Whatever the reasons for the anticipated shortfall, though, it would mean that the cost of promised benefits would outstrip revenues, for Medicare in 2019 and for Social Security retirement by 2042. The figures are staggering, with estimates of the forecasted deficit of unfunded obligations totaling more than $50 trillion over the next seventy-five years. Additionally, the ten-year cost projections of the new Medicare prescription drug benefit for elderly people has a wide gap. Medicare could be on the verge of collapse in the coming years because of the new drug program. Estimates by the CBO put the cost of the program at $395 million from 2004 to 2013, but those could soar to at least $1 trillion over that decade.

While these actuarial estimates are not destiny, the report urges lawmakers to consider raising payroll taxes by 15.5 percent or reducing benefits by 13 percent or both. If nothing is done in the not-too-distant future, a 50 percent increase from today's payroll tax rate will be required.

But does this mean that politicians from both parties will be eager to reach an agreement that calls for changes while the system is still solvent? Is there a *real* fiscal crisis in Social Security retirement programs?

One driver of the politically charged debate is Alan Greenspan, chairman of the Federal Reserve Board for close to two decades, who has urged Congress to cut benefits in order to fully cover the 77 million members of the Baby Boom Generation who will be approaching retirement age over the next 15 years. Current spending on the programs amounts to approximately 7 percent of America's GDP, but that will jump to 12 percent by 2030.

Greenspan and the trustees for Medicare and Social Security moved the topic to center stage in earlier federal budgetary discussions. In the 2004 election year, mature voters were especially aware of these issues. Social Security provides at least half the income for almost two-thirds of the older population (Social Security Administration, 2005). Seasoned older voters are expressing some consternation as they see their retirement incomes slowly evaporate. Despite the congressional gridlock of the 1990s which prevented much action, politicians are beginning to take notice of this situation, because slightly more than 70 percent of citizens age 65–74 years voted in the 2000 election compared to 36 percent of voters 18–24 years (Jamieson, Shin, and Day, 2002).

There is also growing outrage among the aging middle class at their dwindling IRAs and 403(b) accounts. This is important because some experts suggest that half of Americans working today have no employee pension coverage. All told, out of 294 million Americans (U.S. Census Bureau, 2004a) the beneficiary population who received retirement, survivors, and disability benefits in 2004 amounted to almost 47 million people (Social Security Administration, 2005).

Sometimes lost in the political rhetoric are the consequences of long-term insolvency and unsustainability of the system on future generations of retirees, the so-called Generations X and Y, many of whom will be of Hispanic, African American, and Asian ancestry. There is compelling evidence of large racial and ethnic inequities in wealth. Neither the average older black nor older Mexican American household has any financial assets at all.

To help understand the magnitude of the problem, analyses of the University of Michigan's Health and Retirement Study (HRS) and the Survey of Assets and Health Dynamics among the Oldest-Old (AHEAD) by the National Institute on Aging reveal the financial status of individuals in midlife and beyond: (1) The typical household of persons over 70 has less than $9,000 in financial (liquid) assets (not stratifying by race or ethnicity). Among households of the very old in the AHEAD study, the racial and ethnic disparities in financial assets is staggering.

Non-Hispanic whites report $15,586 and African Americans and Hispanics report no liquid assets at all. African Americans and Mexican Americans 51–61 years old will have fewer assets to draw on for long-term care when they reach their seventies and eighties than people currently in that age group. Mean household wealth of middle-aged non-Hispanic whites is a little over $250,000 compared to $71,587 for African Americans and $79,658 for Hispanics.

The data also reveal that, throughout the life course, single women have far lower incomes than either married women or single men, and this pattern persists into old age. As Table 8.2 demonstrates, minority women are at a particular financial disadvantage as they near retirement age. Non-Hispanic black and Hispanic women have lower earnings, lower savings rates, fewer assets, and less extensive pension coverage than non-Hispanic white peers. In addition, other HRS study results indicate that the situation appears to be worse for minority women, for whom marital disruption is increasing and for whom marriage has never been a route to wealth. In the HRS data, Mexican American, other Hispanic, and non-Hispanic black women were far more likely than non-Hispanic whites to experience a reduction in their household income and net worth as the result of losing a husband during the study period. Being black or Hispanic coupled with marital dissolution exaggerates income and wealth inequality. The HRS and AHEAD results also suggest that assuring their financial security will become a greater challenge for minority women in decades to come as norms related to marriage change and if their employment prospects deteriorate (Angel and Angel, 2006; Smith, 1997).

When Social Security was first introduced in 1935, it changed the economic situation of the elderly population and dramatically reduced the number of Americans over 65 living in poverty, from 35 percent in 1935 to less than 11 percent in 2003. More than seven decades after the program's initiation, a significant proportion of elderly women rely on Social Security alone to survive. This highly vulnerable group consists disproportionately of blacks, Hispanics, and immigrants. They earned low wages as workers, spent fewer years in the workforce than did men their age, were more likely to work part-time than full-time when they did work, lack access to private pensions, and had little opportunity to save and invest for retirement. Without Social Security, the total poverty rate among aged beneficiaries would be 67 percent for blacks and 47 percent for whites (Social Security Administration, 2005).

Of course, the overriding issue is whether all elderly Americans will have enough to live on during their latter years. The impact of the enormous potential Social Security deficit on personal retirement security could be devastating. What

TABLE 8.2
Weighted Descriptive Characteristics for Women, by Race and Ethnicity

Demographic	Mexican	Other Hispanic	Non-Hispanic Black	Non-Hispanic White
Age	55.2	55.6	55.6	55.8
Education				
Less than high school	72.5%	54.2%	40.2%	19.3%
High school	17.7%	18.8%	31.5%	43.9%
More than high school	9.8%	27.0%	28.3%	36.8%
Foreign-born	41.7%	65.3%	5.6%	5.4%
Family structure				
Married	65.2%	62.6%	43.9%	74.8%
Partnered	2.8%	0.1%	2.1%	1.6%
Divorced/separated	17.9%	26.4%	29.3%	13.0%
Widowed	10.7%	6.2%	17.1%	7.9%
Never married	3.4%	3.8%	7.6%	2.7%
Number of people in household	3.5%	3.1%	2.9%	2.4%
Economic well-being				
Total household net worth	$87,506.28	$165,985.78	$63,508.27	$262,251.28
Total household income	22,562.98	29,881.18	27,205.71	49,679.38
Earnings	16,173.74	21,740.96	21,343.23	35,206.40
Government transfers	682.46	809.78	937.67	720.91
Pensions and annuities	593.90	2,470.40	1,499.52	2,699.61
Social Security Retirement	666.84	443.22	583.81	835.64
SSI and Disability	629.53	670.77	770.37	542.79
Unemployment and Worker's Compensation	531.51	633.19	225.99	297.72
Other household income	1,256.85	847.40	694.60	2,724.29
Household capital income	2,028.13	2,265.47	1,150.51	6,652.02
Covered by private insurance	37.6%	45.6%	58.2%	74.4%
Unweighted n	318	208	984	4,156

Source: Data from Health and Retirement Study, Wave 1 (1992), as reported in Juster and Suzman, 1995.

is not clear is when Congress will decide to give the issue the serious attention it deserves.

THE FACE OF THE FUTURE WORKFORCE

What are the policy options for public involvement in retirement security in the United States? The deliberations must begin with an assumption that the support of elderly people comes from current resources. The debates over how much elderly people are entitled to will increase in the future, as the Baby Boom Generation, which has been imbued with a desire for a high-quality life, enters the later years of life. In elaborating these issues we examine the decrease in the number of employed people compared to elderly Social Security recipients. The implications of this ratio affects overall economic productivity, because more money will go to consumption rather than investment.

When Social Security was introduced, in the 1930s, there were fifty working individuals for every retiree. At that time, retirement was a luxury; most people could not afford to stop working. Social Security changed that fact. After Social Security was enacted, the program cut the poverty rate among elderly people from 35 percent to less than 11 percent—a two-thirds decrease. More than six decades later, about half of elderly Americans (about 15 million) still depend solely on Social Security to survive, especially members of ethnic minorities (62 percent of elderly blacks and 61 percent of elderly Latinos compared with 49 percent of elderly non-Hispanic whites) (Angel and Angel, 2006).

Today more than half of working men take advantage of the early retirement provisions of Social Security that allow them to leave the labor force at 62; many more women are working later than age 62. The number of active workers supporting each retiree has shrunk to three, and by the time the Baby Boom Generation retires that number will be down to two. That is truly a world we have not seen before. We dare not enter it with blinders on. As a society, we must begin understanding and planning for the huge demographic change we are about to face.

Even with Social Security benefits, certain elderly groups remain in poverty or precariously close to it. This highly vulnerable group, consisting disproportionately of blacks, Hispanics, and female heads of households, is expected to grow substantially over the next several years. The projected older Latino population will more than double, from approximately 2 million in 2000 to almost 5 million in 2020. By that time, Latinos will have surpassed African Americans as the largest segment of elderly minority Americans. These groups, especially people of Mexican descent, are also those most likely to earn low wages as workers, lack access to private pensions, and have little opportunity to save and invest for their own retirement. As a result, they will rely heavily on Social Security.

Sadly, as a 1997 survey by the Pew Charitable Trusts found, approximately one-third of Latinos who are not poor now fear poverty in old age, compared with one-fifth of non-Latinos (white and black). Providing retirement security for Latinos, especially those Mexican American individuals who come to the United States late in life, will be a major challenge in years to come (Angel, 2003).

POLICY OPTIONS: PUBLIC, PRIVATE, AND COMBINED

Proposed remedies for the problem of Social Security funding include reducing cost of living allowances (COLAs), raising payroll taxes, cutting benefits, and creating private investment accounts. Are the burdens of these reform proposals fairly shared throughout the population? Will the most vulnerable be left even more vulnerable? Is privatization the solution? Unfortunately, there are no easy answers, and each option has drawbacks.

Option 1: Reduce Cost of Living Adjustments

Reducing Social Security COLAs would erode the value of benefits relative to prices over time. This would leave minorities more vulnerable, because they are more likely to rely solely on their Social Security checks to support themselves.

Option 2: Increase Payroll Taxes

Increasing the payroll tax could diminish the economic status of low-income workers and families by extracting a disproportionately large share of income from these workers.

Option 3: Reduce Benefits

Reducing benefits would have serious negative implications for minority re-tirees, because these groups disproportionately rely on Social Security as the sole source of retirement income and often receive lower benefits than other groups. Benefit cuts would need to be applied progressively to avoid overburdening poor elderly retirees.

Option 4: Raise the Eligibility Age

Raising the age at which Social Security can be received could hurt African Americans, because they typically have shorter life spans than white Americans and so would pay into the system for as many years as others, or more, but might not benefit as much.

Option 5: Privately Controlled Retirement Accounts

Privatization is the most dramatic proposal for saving Social Security. The rationale of privatization is that if people invest their money themselves, they will get a higher return than if they invest it with the government. Private investment accounts could reduce poverty protection for low-wage earners because of their risks:

- There are no lifetime, inflation-adjusted benefits.
- Financial payouts depend more on the number of working years and earnings levels—having less to invest means lower benefits upon retirement. Minorities on average earn less than the majority, so less money would go into their investment accounts.
- People with low incomes will have to depend on the stock market and investment performance for retirement security, because they are unlikely to have substantial savings accounts or pensions outside of Social Security. Their retirement standard of living would depend on how the money is invested and the amount of income contributed to their personal account.
- Private plans would create a two-tiered system and affect the distribution of wealth in the country, widening the gap between the rich and the poor.
- Low-income workers have limited experience with and exposure to private investments and financial institutions in general, and therefore lack investment expertise.

If Congress makes big cuts to retirees across-the-board, African Americans and Hispanics would be particularly hard hit. According to James Smith, a senior economist at RAND Corporation, Social Security income is almost the only wealth for these retirees. In a RAND study of HRS participants (Smith, 1997), white households headed by someone aged 51 to 61 years had an average of $17,300 in financial assets, enough to live on for about six months in an emergency. In contrast, African American households had just $400 of financial assets and Hispanics only $150.

If Congress further raises the retirement age, the Social Security system will tilt even more against Hispanics and African Americans. Despite paying into the system their whole lives, African American males have an average life span of 65 years. Black male children born in 1990 are projected to live to 67, while white males are projected to live to age 73. Increasing the retirement age may exacerbate a system that takes payroll taxes from African American and Hispanic workers without a better than even chance of ever seeing the retirement benefits of it. We must also ask whether the burdens of these proposed reforms are fairly distributed throughout the population or whether some groups will suffer more of their negative consequences than others?

Will the most vulnerable women be left even more vulnerable? Currently, the Social Security retirement program is based on a male-breadwinner model that assumes that a woman's retirement security will be assured by marriage to a male who has a pension and is able to save for retirement. The fact that black and Hispanic males have never been able to save for retirement or to amass assets makes this model less appropriate for minority women. The failure of the male-breadwinner model and the fact that women in general, and minority women in particular, accumulate fewer assets on their own than men and are less likely to have a private retirement plan means that they are highly vulnerable to poverty in old age. The average woman gains relatively more than men from Social Security; the Social Security benefit structure favors dependents and lower earners, most of whom are female or children. But profound changes in labor force participation rates and marital behavior have ended the male-breadwinner model of retirement security, calling for future cohorts of working-age women to manage their retirement income. For example, because women live longer than men, they are more likely to be widowed or divorced in later life. Consequently, minority women who outlive their husbands or do not qualify for their survivor benefits may suffer a substantial drop in economic status.

Besides reforming Social Security, Congress needs to look at efforts to improve access to private pensions and increased personal savings and investment by low-wage women employees. Social Security alone cannot effectively prevent poor female workers from becoming poor retirees. The rationale of private investment accounts is that if people invest their money themselves, they will get a higher return than if they have it with the government. Private investment accounts could reduce poverty protection for low-wage female workers because women on average earn less than men and work fewer years, so less money would go into their investment accounts. According to a decade-old study by the General Accounting Office, however, women tend to be more conservative investors than are men (General Accounting Office, 1996). If the market performs well, their cautious investing could leave them even further behind the retirement incomes drawn by men (Trout, 1997).

Finally, proposals to privatize Social Security could hurt women whose marriage ends in divorce when they are in their fifties because none of the proposed investment plans seeks to provide monthly payments to an ex-spouse. Splitting the investment account at divorce would help the ex-spouse at the worker's expense, yet this would not guarantee the same income that Social Security currently pays. Moreover, spouses get no income guarantees if a worker dies (because the retired worker can take out money as needed, in a lump sum, or as a lifetime annuity).

HEALTH CARE INSECURITY

The same demands on Social Security that have already or will soon dramatically increase are also affecting our social medical programs, Medicare and Medicaid. Since 1965, when Medicare was introduced, the rate in the growth of expenditures for medical care under this program has increased dramatically (Moon, 2000). In addition, during the 1990s, Medicaid expenditures for hospital and physician services as well as long-term care to elderly poor people have also grown dramatically. Today, although single women and their children comprise the majority of *recipients* of Medicaid, disabled persons and elderly persons in long-term care account for the majority of Medicaid *expenditures* (Harris, 2005).

Unfortunately, there is little reason to imagine that any implicit upper limit to the growth in medical care expenditures for elderly people exists. Although officially defined poverty is low among elderly people now, the retirement incomes of many older Americans are modest; and many, especially among minority elderly people, find their share of payments for medical care burdensome. Currently, Medicaid provides coverage to only a third of the older population in poverty (Harris, 2005). Those not covered by Medicaid must rely on Medicare alone, managing somehow to cover the premiums, deductibles, and copayments out of current income, or they must do without services. Providing supplemental coverage to all poor elderly Americans, through either Medicaid or some other program, would add greatly to aggregate health care costs and divert money from other uses. For the foreseeable future, therefore, the forces propelling the growth in health care costs, including advances in technology and an aging population, will make it difficult, and perhaps impossible, to contain the growth in health care expenditures.

In addition, although studies show that over 80 percent of disabled elderly people can rely on someone for help if they become infirm, the contemporary family is often stretched to the limit in providing such support: single mothers who must raise children alone, couples in which both husband and wife work and so are not available for direct caregiving, and children who have moved away from their parents' community or who have no siblings and cannot handle the financial or caregiving burden alone (Angel and Angel, 1997). The costs of family caregiving are enormous. Studies have pointed to the economic loss to employers—between $11.4 and $29 billion per year—due to employee hours lost to family caregiving. Female caregivers suffer an average loss of $660,000 in wage wealth over their work lives. Over a lifetime, the lost Social Security retirement income averages $25,494.

Many policy makers are worried that Medicare may not be able to provide the level of services that the 40 million frail and disabled Medicare beneficiaries need today. As noted earlier, some observers have begun to question the appropriateness of devoting such a large share of public resources to elderly Medicare beneficiaries (Holahan and Palmer, 1988). Again, elderly people comprise 12.4 percent of the U.S. population but they account for more than 50 percent of federal social welfare spending (Congressional Budget Office, 2000). And, contrary to popular belief, the elderly population consumes far more in lifetime benefits than they contributed in payroll taxes (Myles, 2002).

It is even more important to recognize that Baby Boomers will inevitably demand the same level of benefits as they approach retirement. In fact, experts predict that Medicare may hemorrhage sooner than we thought, given the aging of the population, the soft economy, and the soaring medical care costs. The numbers are staggering. Medicare spending will begin outstripping tax revenue in 2016. Right now, Medicare accounts for 12 percent of federal spending. That budget will triple over the next 30 years, jumping from $233 billion to $694 billion to cover 69 million older adults over the age of 65. However, the ratio of workers to Medicare beneficiaries will drop from 4.0 workers today to 2.3 in 2030. This means that the financial gap—the total Medicare outlays relative to tax receipts and premiums—will widen from $51 billion in 2000 to more than $300 billion by 2030, becoming a burden to the next generation.

Aside from escalating governmental expenditures, our current health care financing regime for seniors often leaves them vulnerable to out-of-pocket costs not covered by traditional Medicare supplemental plans. These include prescription drugs, long-term care, physician fees, and other outpatient costs. Beneficiaries spent almost one-fifth of their annual personal income for health care services last year, at a cost of $2,580 per person. What's worse is that the annual Part B premium, the component that covers physician services, is projected to cost $1,320 per enrollee by 2011.

True, Medicare has reduced racial and ethnic disparities in access to health care, but it has not eliminated them, especially for low-income groups and Hispanic elders. Four in ten Medicare beneficiaries have incomes below 200 percent of poverty. Older Hispanic Americans are particularly susceptible to spiraling medical care costs in later life.

Recent research based on the National Institute on Aging's Longitudinal Study of Elderly Hispanics shows serious deficiencies in health care coverage among many older Mexican Americans, resulting, in part, from a lack of private "Medigap" supplemental coverage (Angel, Angel, and Markides, 2002). The greater reliance among Mexican American seniors on Medicare alone means that they may lack access to the full repertoire of needed services and supports. For those with low incomes and no private supplemental medical insurance, what seems to a middle-class person like a moderate individual contribution may be more than a poorer individual or couple can afford.

It may be unrealistic to imagine that we could develop a chronic care system in which any elder could receive all of the services available to the most affluent retirees. On the other hand, it is a moral imperative to assure that our system of elder care does not leave older Americans with inadequate coverage.

In general, Americans today enjoy the longest and healthiest lives in human history. Older people surviving at age 80 can expect to live another seven to ten years. But, recent improvements in longevity and health depend on the availability of effective and often extremely expensive drugs, which may run more than $2,000 per month for an elderly household. The fact that Medicare now provides some prescription drug coverage may offset these high costs for some families. Nonetheless, even with these Medicare benefits, many elderly persons, especially the near-poor, are only one serious illness away from impoverishment.

Because the cost of acute and long-term care for elderly people accounts for the lion's share of the growth in social welfare expenditures, it is important that Americans across generations focus heavily on Medicare financing reform. To avoid the excessive financial burden on the younger population, changes to the Medicare program should be based on the following guiding principles:

1. *Universal social insurance.* The availability of Medicare to all elderly people regardless of income. A means-tested program in which benefits would be taxed or where premiums would be scaled relative to personal income would undermine popular support of the program.

2. *Medicare payroll taxes must not be increased.* If those who are currently old consume a disproportionate share of aggregate wealth and draw even moderately on their children's incomes, the long-term consequences for overall economic vitality may be serious.

3. *Medicare must provide subsidies for low-income elderly persons.* The current retirement income of low-income older adults must be offset with a government safety net, such as Medicaid and Medicare. The greater reliance among seniors on Medicare alone means they may lack access to the full repertoire of needed services. For those with low incomes and no private supplemental medical insurance, what seems like a moderate individual contribution to some may be more than another Medicare beneficiary or

couple can afford. For this reason, it is important that poorer families have the information they need about state assistance programs that help pay Medicare health care costs, known as Medical Savings Programs. Five programs may pay Medicare premiums, deductibles, and coinsurance amounts for eligible low-income Medicare beneficiaries. The most generous one is the Qualified Medicare Beneficiaries, which pays the Medicare Part A and B premiums, deductibles, and coinsurance.

4. *Medicare services must be appropriately rationed.* Health care costs are increasing more rapidly than wages. Because of the impressive gains in life expectancy, older adults are spending their seventies, eighties, nineties, and beyond with fewer disability-free years. Limit the amount of costs devoted to life-sustaining procedures at a time when quality of life may be debatable. Alternatively, privatizing catastrophic coverage, while unfair to those who could not purchase a private insurance plan, would reduce the burden on the young population.

5. *Adequate reimbursement.* Analysts have argued that providers caring for older Medicare recipients should be appropriately compensated based on the nature, type, and scope of service. Federal rules covering reimbursement for medical care under Medicare and Medicaid should determine the exact cost of covering labor-intensive services such as those received in a geriatric primary care setting, to keep people out of nursing homes.

Medicare's success over the past 35 years must be sustained and extended, if only for the simple reason that administrative costs average only 2 percent of program outlays. Compare that to almost 25 percent for the small group private insurance market. Whether Congress and other public leaders will commit themselves to finding ways to improve and strengthen Medicare as a federal program that guarantees affordable, high-quality, comprehensive health care to all entitled seniors as well as to persons with disabilities is as yet unknown. It is clear that Medicare financing reform should be an urgent social policy priority.

Finally, recoveries from nursing home residents' estates could offset Medicaid long-term care program costs (Arling, Buhaug, Hagan, and Zimmerman, 1991). The state typically uses two methods to recover the cost of benefits. This process of repayment consists of filing claims in probate court for the period when the Medicaid recipient was in long-term care—whether at home, in the community, or in a nursing home—and, if appropriate, filing a lien on the deceased person's house. Between 14 and 35 percent of those admitted to nursing homes as private-pay patients spend down to Medicaid. As Chapter 7 discussed, this is a process whereby a person runs out of, divests, or transfers to others his or her assets and becomes eligible for Medicaid (Short et al., 1992). Among those who enter nursing homes as private-pay patients, nearly 70 percent reach the poverty level after only three months; 90 percent do so within one year.

In Texas, for instance, this means that an unmarried person must have no more than 300 percent of the Supplemental Security Income (SSI) benefit, which in 2001 was $1,593 in income each month and no more than $2,000 in resources. In many cases, however, persons need a nursing facility but exceed the income threshold. To alleviate some of the hardship of this situation, the state established a new kind of entity, called a Miller Trust or Qualifying Income Trust, to keep a potential Medicaid long-term care recipient's income from exceeding the $1,593 limit (Texas Office of the Secretary of State, 2004). The law protects only income, not assets. In 2003, the state enacted a new statute, which requires the Texas Health and Human Services Commission to establish rules in compliance with the Medicaid estate recovery program to request some of the Medicaid expenditures spent on behalf of the deceased Medicaid beneficiary (Texas Administrative Code, 1995).

IMPLICATIONS AND CONCLUSIONS

Old people are consuming an ever-larger fraction of our economic pie (Peterson, 1999). Because Social Security payments were indexed to the rate of inflation as it was in the 1960s, poverty among elders, at least as it is defined in terms of the official U.S. government poverty level, has decreased dramatically. Indeed, poverty today is concentrated among families with young children.

This social trend will cause the nation to reconsider its old-age entitlement programs, because the social contract between generations faces significant structural changes. Because never before have so many people in the United States lived so long and because the shrinking size of families means that the proportion of elderly people is growing faster than the number of younger potential caretakers, young people now can expect to spend more years caring for an elderly parent than raising their own children. Changes in family structure, including increases in childless couples, single-parent families, and delayed childbearing, alter the traditional patterns of intergenerational care. The growth of the welfare state in the last century has forced generations to compete for the entitlement programs that provide social and economic assistance. Children are poor because their parents are poor, and their parents are poor because of market forces that have nothing to do with elders. With the doubling of the elderly population over the next thirty years, we have no choice but to address the need for change in both Social Security and Medicare (Angel and Angel, 2006).

Today we still have a relatively small number of retirees compared to a relatively large number of working-age citizens. This is about to change, perhaps permanently. The Baby Boom Generation is poised to begin getting Social Security benefits in less than a decade. At the same time, longevity is increasing, perhaps faster than official projections note. The twin pressures of increasing longevity and Baby Boomers' retirement will result in an increase in the portion of elderly from about 12 percent of the nation's population in 2003 to 20–24 percent by 2040. Today's preschoolers, who will be working-age taxpayers when that time comes, may find it a struggle to finance Social Security, Medicare, and large portions of Medicaid—the chief income security and health insurance supports for elderly Americans—if other changes are not made.

Because our economic pie is finite, will there be a potential conflict between generations that will result from having to pay for the welfare of old people at the expense of the needs of children and young adults? The aging of the Baby Boom Generation will create a politically powerful gerontocracy which will demand the rewards of their own efforts by drawing on the resources of a small, increasingly minority, and potentially less productive younger population (Angel and Angel, 2006). Current deficit health care spending for the support of older persons will only exacerbate the situation in decades to come.

This situation of a progressively aging population will dramatically affect how parents across the economic spectrum deal with retirement savings, spending, and inheritance. Undoubtedly, the family of the twenty-first century, more than any other institution, will play a greater role in defining private transfers and the quality of the relationship with heirs, whether it be with children, relatives, friends, or charitable organizations. Indeed, the family may provide the only reliable support available to future generations.

People accept sacrifice if they feel that it is the right thing to do and if they feel that they will eventually reap some reward. Few of us object to paying for Social Security and Medicare, because our parents need these programs and some day we will need them. What we must do today is find some balance between the expectation that individuals will take responsibility for their own retirement and long-term care and the expectation that the state will provide a safety net for those who cannot care for themselves.

Although we cannot offer simple solutions to the problems that the coming decades will bring, we can offer the observation that those solutions exist and that as a society we can find them. Any solutions will require a spirited bipartisan debate among politicians and constituents that addresses the multifaceted challenges facing our society and our future. It is for these reasons that the last chapter is dedicated to a summary of the financial issues and diverse challenges we face in the coming decades, and poses key research questions related to inheritance that deserve critical attention.

CHAPTER NINE

Summary and New Directions for Research

In this chapter I highlight major recent research findings about intergenerational gift giving and bequests and propose a research agenda with fertile questions and issues to be addressed by researchers and policy makers in the coming decades. The evidence intermingled throughout this book helps open new windows to understanding the ways we think about our gift-giving behaviors in late life and their effect on our personal legacy. But, in many cases, the data in this study raise more questions than they answer. Set out below is a set of issues that will call for a conversation among family members, public officials, and interest groups, to address the myriad family-relations matters associated with retirement security in aging America. Toward that end, I list some thought-provoking questions to stimulate discussion.

This study took me on a personal journey of discovery that consisted of different approaches to the intended and unintended consequences of gift giving and wealth transfers in middle-class American families. A constellation of factors in the United States—demographic, political, legal, economic, ideological, and health—will affect inheritance decisions and behavior, and family practice in the future. As Chapter 2 discussed, political and legal aspects of gift giving can increase or decrease a family's access to different types of retirement income and wealth (private or public). In traditional societies, the transfer of property from one generation to the next was governed by common law and social practice. Widows and adult children shared property according to prescribed norms. Today the transfer of property, like so much else in modern life, is not governed by established norms and practices but is left to the individual, within the bounds of relevant laws. Increasingly, decisions must be made about dividing property among half-siblings and between different families with a common parent. For this reason, leaving a legacy in the twenty-first century will, in large part, evolve around family values learned in childhood and on the beliefs and attitudes toward financial exchanges one develops as one matures.

Despite these findings, efforts to understand the effects of public policies designed to influence individual-level accumulation of wealth often fail to assess the economic policies of aging in the larger context of the goals of other social welfare programs. As yet, governmental proposals, such as the Pension Protection Act, which aims to protect employees' pensions, and its implications for health care of older adults and their heirs, have not been fully grasped by advocates and lawmakers. Baby Boomers are not a monolithic group, and the age heterogeneity among this birth cohort has ramifications for future support of health entitlements such as Medicare and catastrophic coverage. While these changes in the law will shift more of the burden to workers, employers will also bear a potential cost. Consequently, the increasing regulation of pensions could lessen a corporation's willingness to sponsor traditional pensions and could diminish future employer support of any retirement benefit proposals.

Lessons can be learned, as shown in Chapter 3, from the current institutional regimes of pension programs in industrialized nations such as Sweden, France, and Italy, which are undergoing dramatic demographic change in caring for their elderly citizens. These nations mirror aging trends in the United States and portend serious problems and challenges for the future of economic security for generations to come if action is not taken to strengthen the state's obligations to families across the life course. Although the state is often viewed as the safety net for older people in the developed world, increasingly many Americans are turning to family for support, as they enter their retirement years without any private wealth or substantial assets or income.

What emerges from the research is recognition that the family dynamics associated with "gift giving" in late life are complex. The complexities inherent in the decision-making process are deeply textured, and it is difficult to unlock the personal meaning and perspectives of familial money exchange. What is not to be disputed is that the personal motivations underlying intergenerational transfers are anchored in people's histories. The extent to which early childhood experiences can color an individual's view of gift giving in later life is stunning. The voices of older adults and their adult children display their deepest feelings and emotions regarding their childhood experiences with family money.

In my research, most families stated that they see leaving and receiving inheritances as an act of love from one generation to the next. People believe that the right way to handle their estate, however modest it may be, is to tell their children the reasons for passing down their assets, and what role they expect them to play in maintaining the family's values. When planning a will, most parents expect to divide their estate equally among their children, in part because they do not want to show favoritism or cause any resentment among family members.

However, the data reveal a picture that is more complicated and nuanced. It is not uncommon for people to assume and believe that the way they think about gift giving is well intended. But what is unearthed in the narratives of gift-giving behavior suggests that motives are fraught with problems when it comes time to dividing an estate, even a modest one. Family strains are apparent when parents did not engage their children or other relatives in discussions. The preponderance of the data shows that when older family members do not openly share their feelings, specifically regarding expectations of gifts and bequests, it can result in serious long-term consequences for relationships within the family. While the majority of elderly parents feel confident enough in their decisions to inform their children of their wishes, wants, and desires, many of the people whom I interviewed felt uncomfortable holding such conversations. Quite often, either nonaction or denial was the response instead. Although financial honesty is the best policy, for many older people denial can be an effective coping mechanism, at least in the short run. Denial often leads to delays in preparing a will, speaking to adult children, and planning for one's own death. In the long run, however, avoiding the decision-making process can lead to ill will among family members and unnecessary problems and expenses in distribution of an estate.

Although making sure that all important family members are informed of estate planning helps avoid trouble after one has died, many respondents had not raised this issue with their families; indeed, they had not even thought about it. But, misunderstandings about the distribution of family wealth and belongings occur frequently, often alienating siblings from one another. Such deep-seated negative feelings are seldom anticipated by parents, especially those who avoid planning.

THE DEMOGRAPHY OF GIFT GIVING IN LATE LIFE

The results of this study show that how much older adults expect to pass on to the next generation and their grandchildren varies greatly by social background, family beliefs, and birth cohort. Our study confirms what previous researchers observed in gift-giving behavior across generations. Not surprisingly, socioeconomic status plays a critical role in when gifts are made, if for no other reason than it dictates how much a person can afford to give. Events also influence giving. When all is well, giving is more possible, more generous, and can go as planned, but an elderly parent may end up having medical needs that obviate his or her capacity to give, if steps were not taken before the financial exigency.

The other most significant social structural factors generating different expectations and obligations in gift-giving behavior include parent's age, offspring's age and gender, and offspring's needs. These factors taken together make a significant difference in gift-giving decisions and behavior throughout the adult life course. It became clear from our research that a child's economic situation trumped all other factors when it came to inter vivos transfers. Those children who needed financial assistance were more often than not provided with resources to the best of the parent's ability, sometimes with strings attached; but more times than not, the transfers were considered gifts as opposed to loans. Equal treatment of children can be difficult when one has done significantly better than another. The ability to give to a child, especially when he or she is in financial trouble, is also a reflection of a parent's own success. The fair distribution of assets may not be easily calculated, owing to children's changing circumstances and their needs for assistance (Gruber, 2003).

Another complicating factor is that the parent is increasingly becoming the one who needs financial assistance. Crossing the line from support provider to needy elderly parent is fraught with difficulties in many instances. Often, embarrassment, pride, or a determination to remain self-reliant keeps the financial line in the sand drawn between a parent and her or his children.

The age-related differences defined in terms of birth cohort revealed in our study were significant. These data suggest a generational shift in inheritance. Traditional attitudes toward gift giving are changing. Significant demographic forces are redefining the expectations and obligations associated with retirement behavior in general and how people perceive their security in late life, with respect to private pensions, savings, housing assets, and Social Security, all of which undeniably affect the relationship between birth cohorts, between the state and the family, and between older parents and adult children, in particular.

SHOULD WOMEN WORRY ABOUT THEIR RETIREMENT?

Gender dimensions also emerged in the research. The transfer of estates from one generation to the next has become more complicated for women in particular. Baby Boomers are now set to retire in record numbers, beginning in 2007 when the first group turns age 60; the issue is becoming more salient as changes in social insurance programs like Social Security and Medicare are debated in Congress. Both adult children and elderly parents are taking stock of how inheritance may affect their retirement security, given rising health care costs and vanishing private pension plans.

As elderly parents, the majority of whom are women, grow older, they tend to focus on their financial security, but women are more likely to be without a safety net. As older women reach deep old age, the mideighties and later, a potential loss of executive functioning can lead to problems in handling money, if steps have not been taken to protect the economic well-being of the very old person.

Women in general, and widows in particular, of the Silent Generation spoke in this study about their unconditional love for their children, including disappointments with children who were still dependent on them after leaving home, and expressed concern about balancing what they intended to pass on to their children relative to what they could afford, given their health situation and contemplating their need for long-term care. Men, on the other hand, tended to respond in a more strategic or instrumental manner, with fewer emotions guiding their decisions regarding long-term care plans. Many elderly respondents felt a family obligation to speak to their children in advance, before a medical crisis occurred, about their bequest intentions. They explained what they hoped to leave to their children and why. As one respondent put it, at the end of the day, this is one of the best gifts an elderly parent can give a child or other loved one.

Baby Boomer women rarely mentioned any concerns about their finances. For single Baby Boomers, the focus on financial literacy was important, although discussing the gift-giving decision-making process seemed difficult. Married women often left financial decisions, like whether to invest, to their husbands. Married men usually assumed the traditional role in family regarding retirement planning. But, what the research results also suggest is that assuring the financial security of future generations will become a greater challenge for women as norms related to marriage change and as fewer jobs in the service sector provide benefit packages that include a retirement plan.

Currently, the Social Security retirement program is based on a male-breadwinner model that assumes that a woman's retirement security will be assured by marriage to a man who has a pension and is able to save for retirement (Herd, 2005). The fact that black and Hispanic men have faced serious barriers to the accumulation of assets and have often spent their working years in jobs with low wages and no retirement plans makes this model less appropriate for minority women (Herd, 2006). The failure of the male-breadwinner model and the fact that women in general, and minority women in particular, accumulate fewer assets on their own than men do means that women are highly vulnerable to poverty in old age. This is especially true in the event of widowhood.

The changes noted above clearly call for the end of the male-breadwinner model of retirement security. Future cohorts of working-age women will manage their own retirement income sources. Because of the labor force disadvantages they face, the situation of low-wage service sector workers and the unemployed and underemployed requires special attention. For this reason, any changes to be made to the present Social Security system will need to take these vulnerabilities into account.

Therefore, proposals aimed at cutting benefits as opposed to generating revenue are problematic if the program aims to protect minority group widows from outliving their savings (Kotlikoff and Burns, 2005). The powerful AARP and many Democrats state that the main reason for avoiding benefit cuts is clear: Social Security represents a major pillar of minority widows' old-age security, making up a major portion of their retirement income, and any reductions in their monthly benefits could make their lives worse. Most significantly, both liberal and centrist Democrats alike argue that the program helps keep low-income minority women from falling into poverty because it enables retirement income to keep up with inflation and to be protected over their lifetime from financial risks (Aaron and Reischauer, 2001).

In addition to reforming Social Security, efforts to improve access to private pensions and increased personal savings and investment by low-wage women employees are needed (Herd, 2005). Some critics suggest that Social Security alone cannot effectively guarantee the old-age security of low-wage workers. At the top of the list is the privatization proposal of the president's 2005 Commission to Strengthen Social Security, although the idea was eventually dropped by the Bush administration. The commission recommended creating private investment accounts that would allow people to invest the money themselves. Advocates favor privatization because they believe retirees could get a higher return than when they rely on traditional Social Security. Privatization proponents also support these plans because they feel they would enhance the potential for bequests (Munnell, Sundén, Soto, and Taylor, 2003). Unfortunately, proposals for pension reform are largely irrelevant to workers with no pension coverage, and privatization of Social Security, without other reforms, could only increase the risk for minority workers. Low-income households, especially female-headed families, have limited experience with private investments, such as stock ownership, and with financial institutions in general and therefore lack investment expertise

(Choudhury, 2001–2002). Privatization of the Social Security retirement program would have serious disadvantages for women, in general.

The data demonstrate that old-age economic security of women is greatly affected by race and Hispanic ethnicity. General reforms to public and private retirement systems may well increase the choices available to affluent workers, but they are not likely to increase the economic security of low-wage or minority workers. Targeted programs that focus on the most vulnerable could more directly address the unique needs of older black and Hispanic women, but like targeted programs in general, they run the risk of stigmatizing the recipients and of generating political opposition. Whatever the future holds, public policy focused on old-age economic security cannot ignore gender, race, or ethnicity. As a result, the AARP, the largest interest group representing the concerns of persons age 50 or older, will continue to fervently speak against any reforms that could potentially threaten these entitlements (Schulz and Binstock, 2006). The membership's interest in the protection of Social Security is underscored by a 2005 survey, which found that 40 percent of respondents expect Social Security to be a chief source of income, because employers are increasingly reducing or eliminating private pensions (AARP, 2005).

GENERATIONAL DIFFERENCES:
MONEY MEMORIES AND FAMILY IDEOLOGY

This study challenges the mainstream argument and the consensus among most researchers that structural factors alone account for expectations in gift giving and bequests in the United States. Thinking about how to transfer money from one generation to the next is also associated with the meaning that people attach to money, regardless of their age, income, or child's situation. Historical period and events affect the emotional attitude toward money.

As the family narratives revealed, money carries a different meaning for the Silent Generation. As a result of the Great Depression during the 1930s, they faced the worst economic crisis in contemporary American history. Many elderly people saw their parents retire during the 1920s with a comfortable income but lose everything a decade later as a result of the Great Depression.

The financial devastation experienced by older Americans during the Depression had long-lasting effects on their assessments of risk. That abject loss of economic security resulted in an expression of an inner sense of obligation to be thrifty and to save so as to take care of themselves and to pass on whatever they could to their children.

Today, older Americans expect their Social Security retirement benefits to prevent them from falling into poverty (Mitchell, 2000). Less than 9 percent of the older population lived below the poverty line in 2005. Yet, members of the Silent Generation did not expect to live as long as they have, and concerns about growing costs of health care for disabling chronic conditions like diabetes, heart disease, cancer, and Alzheimer's disease are troubling many elderly people.

Sadly, as health care costs continue to rise and there are plans to reduce or eliminate payments for some medications, the money elders planned to leave to their children may be needed for their own long-term care instead. While a small fraction of older Americans have purchased a private long-term care insurance policy, the need for the rest of them to do so in the future is on the horizon. Ten years ago, the Health Insurance Portability Act of 1996 provided an incentive, through federal tax advantages, to purchase such plans. As Chapter 7 discussed, however, these policies can be costly. Consequently, many older Americans today are faced with two choices: either spend their savings to pay health care costs or long-term care costs or do without. Doing without often requires depending on family members to provide some measure of care. For those with significant assets and income, private long-term care insurance may be worth serious consideration, given that the cost of nursing home care can run as high as $80,000 per year (MetLife, 2002).

That elderly Americans are weighing the costs of health care against doing without that care should not be simply conceded, though (Gustman and Steinmeier, 2003). Baby Boomers are experiencing good health, and the number of active days of life expectancy has steadily increased. This means that elderly people may have fewer needs for medical care and long-term care and therefore are far less concerned about paying for it.

How will AARP mediate the concerns raised by younger Americans, many of whom believe that the Social Security retirement program will not be there when they are older? Garnering younger workers' support of entitlement programs like Medicare and Old-Age Insurance and Survivors benefits is a thorny problem, and it may be a particularly daunting task as children assume a larger financial obligation for older adults. Kotlikoff and Burns (2005) refer to the potential tax burden on many generations to follow as fiscal child abuse. They argue that the recent tax reduction enacted by Congress will only exacerbate what future generations of workers will need to contribute. They predict that many members of Generation X, the cohort of people born between 1965 and 1977, of Generation Y, children born between 1978 and 1990, and people born during the 1990s, Generation D or the Digital Generation, having been unable to participate in these decisions related to tax cuts because they were not of voting age, may oppose any remedies that include substantial increases (as high as a doubling) in payroll taxes to cover promised benefits.

The debate will also be fueled by other actors inside government. For example, former Social Security Administration Commissioner Jo Anne Barnhart, during her term of service (2001–2007), warned workers of the risks of not achieving sustainable Social Security solvency in efforts to educate the next generation of workers about what they can expect to receive in their later years. She underlined the point that, unless measures are taken to strengthen the Medicare and Medicaid trust funds, nearly three-fourths of full benefit commitments will be broken in 2042 due to the exceedingly low dependency ratio of 2.2 workers to every individual receiving benefits (Social Security Administration, 2005). Barnhart's successor, Michael Astrue, has not, as of this writing, weighed in on the debate.

Today, one-third of government funding favors elderly people, yet the issue has largely been neglected by Congress since the debate began thirty years ago (Binstock, 1995). This is in part because Social Security is "the third rail of American politics," a term applied to it by Tip O'Neill, then Speaker of the House, in the early 1980s. Federal lawmakers of all political stripes hesitate to propose reform options for sustaining the system, such as privatization, because they fear that if they do touch the system they will get burned politically. That fear has stymied any progress toward reform.

So, what is a realistic next step? Robert Binstock (2006), a distinguished scholar of political gerontology, finds that the contemporary debate over sharp intergenerational conflict, pitting the young against the old, has lacked focus and cries out for radical solutions. He urges that advocates "reframe the issues [related to generational equity] in terms of strengthening Social Security and Medicare, rather than tearing them down. Banding together its resources, this coalition should launch a sustained media campaign that portrays the aging of the population as a challenge confronting today's elders, boomers, their families, and society —not merely problems in financing Social Security and Medicare" (p. 3).

AN AGENDA FOR FUTURE RESEARCH

The numerous questions raised here provide ample opportunity for others to investigate in more depth the issue of how generational transfers affect not only personal financial legacies but also the larger society's. Family ideologies as they relate to gift giving and inheritance practices will continue to be a topic that deserves much greater attention as the Baby Boom Generation confront their parents' financial affairs in late life. As experts suggest, the difficulties surrounding an elder's death can be exacerbated if family business matters are not taken care of beforehand (Umberson, 2006). Therefore, future studies of gift-giving practices would do well to include new groups of adult children and elderly parents. Combined with larger sample sizes, this research design would ensure that the qualitative data (narratives) would truly reflect the population and diversity of contemporary families. It would also help to develop a better understanding of the role of culture and gift giving in late life within certain social subgroups (e.g., women, ethnic minorities, immigrants). With a larger study sample, tests could be conducted of specific hypotheses regarding differential expectations and obligations for newer cohorts of minority American men and women.

Intergenerational transfers will no doubt affect generations to come. How family relations evolve as old-age dependency increases is a subject that deserves serious reflection. Specifically, how wealth transfers shape sibling relations, whether they positively or negatively affect the relationships of those left behind, and how, is a fertile ground for an enduring research program. It is important to investigate how heirs, particularly siblings, interact with each other after a parent's death and throughout the settling of a parent's estate. Little is known of the quality of kin relations before and immediately following a parent's death and its impact on funeral and wealth management, including insurance and investments.

The generational-equity debate examined by Williamson and colleagues (1999) suggests that studies should examine the dynamics of the myriad actors involved in a serious debate, reaching beyond the usual suspects who have profoundly influenced development of federal social policy of old-age pensions over the last century. These senior movements, including the White House Conferences on Aging and AARP, must evolve to incorporate other interest groups who act on behalf of constituents, including Third Millennium, National Council of La Raza, National Organization for Women, to name just a few. Understanding how these advocacy organizations will represent the growing social welfare needs of aging women, minorities, children, and recent immigrants deserves attention.

Policy studies could concentrate on the array of medical care and social service issues that influence our response to the social policy demands. There is a lack of much-needed information, for instance, on whether age-based health care rationing is a realistic solution to insure Medicare solvency. Other research is needed to estimate the individual and employer costs of health insurance for older workers on the cusp of retirement. Few studies assess the effects of COBRA legislation on individuals' plans for retirement. Gruber and Madrian (1995) observe that Medicare gaps may increase the risk of poor health in late life in spite of COBRA. In the light of this disparity, it would be useful to investigate states' strategies to reduce administrative barriers to promote access to programs for low-income Medicare beneficiaries.

In addition, we need to expand our knowledge of the complexities underlying the many choices at the end of life. Some of the hardest decisions—how to pay for palliative care, how to balance dying and dignity, and how to provide care that meets the personal desires and needs of a loved one with terminal illness—are as of yet poorly understood. The bitter debate over physician-assisted suicide continues without any resolution.

Not surprisingly, some elderly parents are experiencing financial pressures, especially as the result of the ebb and flow of the U.S. economy creating an erratic housing market, outsourcing of U.S. manufacturing jobs to Asia, and a loss in good wages due to the de-skilling of the workforce. In an era of fiscal constraints, family support will take on greater salience, and, as a consequence, researchers will need to uncover the mystery of the new meanings of what finances convey in adult child and parent relationships in the twenty-first century.

Among other issues to explore is the pressing concern certain to consume the attention of elderly parents of at what point in life wealth should be passed on to heirs. Because of the high costs of education, parents will need to ask themselves whether they should consider factoring in tuition costs when determining inheritance or whether children should wait to receive all of their inheritance. Once again, because parents don't want to be a burden to their children and children want their parents to have the best care possible, the tradeoffs in decisions about paying for health care could be problematic without previous family discussion about the various alternatives. In the future, how families weigh the strengths and weaknesses of options in long-term care planning for aging parents and their own situation will be critical in light of the generational equity issues associated with health care spending. For this reason, studies should look in great detail at the effect of age-group differences within the Baby Boomer cohort on retirement planning.

Finally, applied research examining the role of the legal community and the government in helping aging families is a fertile area for research. Much needed empirical information still remains to be produced on how to make informed decisions about one's financial legacy. Understanding the implications of the decision-making process for family well-being could help adult children and their elderly parents enjoy the time spent together during the parents' fourth age and could unravel the complexities and nuances of this critical process.

Exploring the financial implications of family ideologies and wealth transmission for future generations of daughters and sons will require a bold new approach. Social scientists and policy makers will need to consider carefully the situation of ethnicity, marriage, and family from a different point of view in the light of potential changes in old-age welfare policies. All of these factors will influence the decision to accept this challenge.

The research on which this book is based employed both survey and nonquantitative methods. Several factors call for a multimethod approach, including in-depth (semistructured) interviews of adult children and aging parents in addition to detailed quantitative analyses of large-scale nationwide surveys on intergenerational exchanges, bequests, and inheritance. An analytic literature review indicated that a complex set of mechanisms shapes family gift-giving patterns. By employing survey data from the University of Michigan's Health and Retirement Study, sponsored by the National Institute on Aging, and from the Assets and Health Dynamics among the Oldest-Old dataset (AHEAD), an in-depth economic, social, and health database, I could determine the personal value older parents attach to all types of financial giving. At the same time, information about role expectations by the elderly parent could be assessed in some detail. Thus, I chose to develop a case method approach to explore the fabric of emotional relationships and psychic meanings that may be attached to giving. The following summarizes the justification for this analytic approach.

First, inspection of survey data indicates that a complex set of mechanisms shapes family gift-giving patterns. Probing questions, what Howard Schuman refers to as the "random probe," can help to determine people's attitude toward money.

Second, during an in-depth personal interview, the researcher can ask about monetary support received over several years, not simply a short span of time dictated by the survey. The evidence suggests little giving occurs during the course of one year. We asked adult children and parents about any type of financial support the adult child had received since leaving the parents' household. This helped determine whether parent(s) tended to give money at certain times over the life course. For instance, do parents mainly give money to help purchase a new home, for college education, to help the adult child establish a household, or simply when the child is in need? Are inter vivos transfers a functional alternative to inheritance? If so, how do minority families differ from non-Hispanic whites in their definition of wealth transmission and subsequent decision to give substantial gifts?

Finally, a nonquantitative approach made it possible to explore the fabric of emotional relationships and psychic meanings that may be attached to giving. The interview guide was designed to get underneath the numbers revealed in survey research.

I hypothesized that one important factor that may determine giving is the quality of the relationship between the parent and child. Most surveys include questions that inquire about frequency with which the focal adult child speaks to or visits parents, or how good the parent-child relationship is on a scale of 1 to 10. These gauges may not uncover the nuances of the parent-child relationship compared with an in-depth personal interview protocol that queries both parent and child about past conflict over issues such as sibling rivalries, financial assets, and emotional blackmail. Another important variable is how close the adult child has stayed to the parent after leaving home. A child who lived with a step-parent for five years before leaving home may have a very different relationship with that parent than a young child who lived in the parental household for fifteen years or longer.

SAMPLE

To amplify the national (published) data on the role of gift exchanges in defining the new intergenerational contract, an embedded qualitative case study of a multiethnic sample of elderly parents and adult children was conducted on issues related to family gift giving and inheritance. My decision to use this method and to draw a sample of older parents and adult children from the southwestern United States was deliberate. Central Texas is a socioeconomically diverse region and contains one of the largest Mexican American populations in the nation.

To begin the process, a random sample of ninety-four churches located in the city of Austin was selected for potential inclusion in the study. The churches selected for possible inclusion in the study were listed on pages 426–444 of the December 2001 Greater Austin Yellow Pages Book. Fifteen percent of the churches responded to the original mail survey. Follow-up reminder cards were sent to those who had not responded to the first survey.

From this list, church leadership was contacted by letter. The letter described the project goals and invited the congregation to participate in the study. Next, the investigator arranged a meeting to distribute the survey and was available to answer any questions about the study.

Although I did not obtain active written consent, subjects were informed about the study only after permission was received from the church leadership. Participation in the study was strictly voluntary. Potential participants were provided a copy of the questionnaire and asked to complete it at their convenience and to return it in the stamped, self-addressed envelope. The initial survey instrument took approximately 15–20 minutes to complete. Respondents were also given the opportunity to contact the principal investigator with any additional questions about the study. The paper-and-pencil survey contains information about demographic background and attitudes toward inter vivos exchanges, loans, and inheritance practices.

In the second stage of the research, I conducted qualitative interviews with parents 55 years and over and adult children over 18 years old residing in central Texas. The interview guide included a set of questions about their attitudes and expectations toward giving and receiving money in childhood. In addition, personal feelings and information were elicited on perceptions of current exchange and bequest practices. Long-distance telephone interviews were also conducted for focal parents and children who resided outside the state. The final study group was based on a purposive quota sample, which included twenty-five respondent adult children and older parents representing several racial and ethnic groups of African American, European, and Latino/Hispanic ancestry.

With this multicultural matrix, I was able to identify differences based on social characteristics in exchange patterns, the feelings of commitment to performing roles and meeting
filial obligations, and the extent to which economic factors constrain the decision to give
gifts in later life. If the moral obligation outweighs the degree of reciprocity held by parents
and children, then any prior giving or future bequest expectations may not be revealed in
the interviews. Employing this methodology, then, allowed me to capture symbolic ele-
ments of gift giving and bequest motives (reciprocity and altruism) and constraints, if any,
from both the parent's and the child's perspective.

The research posed no risks to the study subjects known at the time the study was
conducted. All information was maintained in strict confidence and no damaging information was collected. Those individuals who wished not to participate in the entire interview
were permitted to discontinue from it. The subjects benefited from the study insofar as
some isolated individuals enjoyed the interaction with the interviewer. The social benefit is
that this project will continue to provide information needed by elder care providers
responsible for guardianship services, money management, and retirement planning.

Appendix B

Questions Used in Semistructured In-Depth Interview

1. What types of gifts did your parents give you growing up?
2. What positive lessons did you learn about money as you grew up?
3. How did your parents handle allowance, if any?
4. What does money and material aid mean to you?
5. What were the biggest conflicts about money, if any?
6. What did you worry about most?
7. Did anyone use money to exert control?
8. Were there any family secrets about money?
9. Were there open discussions about money conflicts?
10. Who was good at handling money?
11. What lessons are you imparting today to your children?
12. What were the biggest conflicts about money?
13. How do you feel about helping family members outside the household with money problems? Do you and your spouse agree?
14. Do you feel that you should talk to your children about their inheritance?
15. Have your children brought up their plans about inheritance? Do you think it is right to raise the issue? Even when stepchildren are involved?
16. Do you believe that you should give each child an equal piece of the pie?
17. Do you think giving gifts before your death is the right thing to do? Do you think it is right to expect certain things from your children in return for inter vivos transfers and inheritance?
18. Do you think you should include grandchildren in your inheritance plan?
19. Are you going to leave anyone else money?
20. How satisfied are you with your life?
21. Before I conclude, I'd just like to get some basic information from you. About how much was your personal income for the past year? Household income? Please include income from all sources, such as wages, salaries, Social Security, retirement benefits, help from relatives, rent from property, and so forth.
22. Please describe whether you own any assets.
23. How much is your house worth?

I'd like to thank you again for all of your help! If you have any questions about anything we discussed, feel free to call me. I will send you a copy of our research findings upon completion of the study.

Bibliography

Aaron, Henry, and Robert Reischauer. 2001. *Countdown to Reform: The Great Social Security Debate*. Washington, DC: Century Foundation Press.

AARP. 1999. *Baby Boomers Envision Their Retirement: An AARP Segmentation Analysis*. Research report by Roper Starch Worldwide. Available at www.aarp.org/research/refe rence/publicopinions/aresearch-import-299.html.

———. 2005. *Social Security 70th Anniversary Survey Report: Trends over Time*. Washington, DC: AARP.

Abel, Andrew B. 2003. "Commentary on 'How Do People Make Gifts and Bequests?'" Pp. 118–126 in *Death and Dollars*, edited by Alicia H. Munnell and Annika Sundén. Washington, DC: Brookings Institution.

Acock, Alan C., and David H. Demo. 1994. *Family Diversity and Well-Being*. Thousand Oaks, CA: Sage Publications.

Aizcorbe, Ana M., Arthur B. Kennickell, and Kevin B. Moore. 2003. "Recent Changes in U.S. Family Finances: Evidence from the 1998 and 2001 Survey of Consumer Finances." *Federal Reserve Bulletin* (January): 1–32.

Altman, Stuart H., Uwe E. Reinhardt, and Alexandra E. Shields, eds. 1998. *The Future U.S. Healthcare System: Who Will Care for the Poor and Uninsured?* Chicago: Health Administration Press.

Altonji, Joseph G., Fumio Hayashi, and Laurence Kotlikoff. 1997. "Parental Altruism and Inter Vivos Transfers: Theory and Evidence." *Journal of Political Economy* 105:1121–1166.

Amato, Paul R., Sandra J. Rezac, and Alan Booth. 1995. "Helping between Parents and Young Adult Offspring: The Role of Parental Marital Quality, Divorce, and Remarriage." *Journal of Marriage and the Family* 57:363–374.

Amenta, Edwin. 2006. *When Movements Matter: The Townsend Plan and the Rise of Social Security*. Princeton: Princeton University Press.

American Bar Association. 2002. Section of Real Property, Probate and Trust Law. Retrieved July 8, 2004, from www.abanet.org/rppt/public/home.html.

American Law Institute. 2007. *American Law Institute–American Bar Association Course of Study: Basic Estate and Gift Taxation and Planning*. Philadelphia: American Law Institute.

Americans for a Fair Estate Tax. 2002. "Public Opinion Poll: Americans Support Reforming, Not Repealing Estate Tax." Retrieved July 7, 2004, from www.responsiblewealth .org/press/2002/americans_support_pr.html.

Anderton, Douglas L., Richard E. Barrett, and Donald J. Bogue. 1997. *The Population of the United States*. New York: Free Press.

Angel, Jacqueline L. 1991. *Health and Living Arrangements of the Elderly*. New York: Garland.

———. 1999. "Helping Families to Navigate the System of Long-term Care Alternatives: The Role of Information Technology." *Journal of Family and Consumer Sciences* 91:116–123.

———. 2001. "Long-term Health Care Reform: Who Is Going to Care for Us?" *Austin American-Statesman*, May 3, A15.

———. 2003. "Devolution and the Social Welfare of Elderly Immigrants: Who Will Bear the Burden?" *Public Administration Review* 63:79–89.

Angel, Jacqueline L., Ronald J. Angel, J. L. McClellan, and Kyriakos S. Markides. 1996. "Nativity, Declining Health, and Preferences in Living Arrangements among Elderly Mexican Americans: Implications for Long-term Care." *The Gerontologist* 36:464–473.

Angel, Jacqueline L., and Dennis P. Hogan. 2004. "Population Aging and Diversity in a New Era." Pp. 128–139 in *Closing the Gap: Improving the Health of Minority Elders in the New Millennium*, edited by Keith E. Whitfield. Washington, DC: Gerontological Society of America.

Angel, Jacqueline L., Maren A. Jiménez, and Ronald J. Angel. 2007. "The Economic Consequences of Widowhood for Older Minority Women." *The Gerontologist* 47:224–234.

Angel, Ronald J., and Jacqueline L. Angel. 1993. *Painful Inheritance: Health and the New Generation of Fatherless Families*. Madison: University of Wisconsin Press.

———. 1997. *Who Will Care for Us? Aging and Long-term Care in America*. New York: New York University Press.

———. 2006. "Diversity and Aging." Pp. 94–110 in *Handbook of Aging and the Social Sciences*, 6th edition, edited by Robert Binstock and Linda George. San Diego, CA: Academic Press.

Angel, Ronald J., Jacqueline L. Angel, Geum-Yong Lee, and Kyriakos S. Markides. 1999. "Age at Migration and Family Dependency among Older Mexican Immigrants: Recent Evidence from the Mexican American EPESE." *The Gerontologist* 39:59–65.

Angel, Ronald J., Jacqueline L. Angel, and Kyriakos S. Markides. 2002. "Stability and Change in Health Insurance among Older Mexican Americans: Longitudinal Evidence from the Hispanic-EPESE." *American Journal of Public Health* 92:1264–1271.

Angel, Ronald J., and Marta Tienda. 1982. "Determinants of Extended Household Structure: Cultural Pattern or Economic Need?" *American Journal of Sociology* 87:1360–1383.

Aquilino, William S., and Khalil R. Supple. 1991. "Parent-Child Relations and Parent's Satisfaction with Living Arrangements When Adult Children Live at Home." *Journal of Marriage and the Family* 35:13–27.

Arling, Greg, Harald Buhaug, Shelley Hagan, and David Zimmerman. 1991. "Medicaid Spenddown among Nursing Home Residents in Wisconsin." *The Gerontologist* 31:174–182.

Arthur, W. Brian, and Geoffrey McNicoll. 1978. "Samuelson Population and Intergenerational Transfers." *International Economic Review* 19:241–246.

Assistant Secretary for Planning and Evaluation. 2005. *Long-Term Growth of Medical Expenditures Public and Private: ASPE Issues Brief.* Washington, DC: U.S. Department of Health and Human Services. From aspe.hhs.gov/health/MedicalExpenditures/index .shtml.

Baker, Dean, and Mark Weisbrot. 1999. *Social Security: The Phony Crisis.* Chicago: University of Chicago Press.

Barer, Barbara M., and Colleen L. Johnson. 1990. "A Critique of the Caregiving Literature." *The Gerontologist* 30:26–29.

Barro, Robert J. 1974. "Are Government Bonds Net Wealth?" *Journal of Political Economy* 82:1095–1117.

Becker, Gary S. 1974. "A Theory of Social Interactions." *Journal of Political Economy* 82:1063–1094.

Bengston, Vern L. 1985. "Generations, Cohorts, and Relations between Age Groups." Pp. 339–368 in *Handbook of Aging and the Social Sciences,* edited by Robert H. Binstock and Ethel Shanas. New York: Van Nostrand Reinhold.

Bengtson, Vern L., and Robert A. Harootyan, eds. 1994. "Generational Linkages and Implications for Public Policy." Pp. 210–234 in *Intergenerational Linkages: Hidden Connections in American Society.* New York: Springer.

Bengtson, Vern L., and Robert E. L. Roberts. 1991. "Intergenerational Solidarity in Aging Families: An Example of Formal Theory Construction." *Journal of Marriage and the Family* 53:856–870.

Benson, Mark J., Joyce Arditti, Julia T. Reguero de Atiles, and Suzanne Smith. 1992. "Intergenerational Transmission: Attributions in Relationships with Parents and Intimate Others." *Journal of Family Issues* 13:450–464.

Bernheim, B. Douglas, and Sergei Severinov. 2000. "Bequests as Signals: An Explanation for the Equal Division." NBER Working Paper No. 7791. Cambridge, MA: National Bureau of Economic Research. Retrieved July 7, 2004 from ideas.repec.org/p/nbr/ nberwo/7791.html.

Bernheim, B. Douglas, Andrei Shleifer, and Lawrence H. Summers. 1985. "The Strategic Bequest Motive." *Journal of Political Economy* 93:1045–1076.

Berry, Brent M. 2001. "Financial Transfers from Parents to Adult Children: Issues of Who Is Helped and Why." Population Studies Center Report No. 01-485. Ann Arbor: University of Michigan.

Binstock, Robert. 1995. "Policies on Aging in the Post–Cold War Era." Pp. 55–90 in *Post–Cold War Policy,* vol. 1, *The Social and Domestic Context,* edited by William Crotty. Chicago: Nelson-Hall Publishers.

———. 2006. "Politics and Policy in Aging: A Political Scientist's Journey." *Aging Today* 27:3–4.

Bipartisan Commission on Entitlement and Tax Reform. 1995. *Report to the President.* Washington, DC: Government Printing Office.

Blaikei, Andrew. 1999. *Ageing and Popular Culture.* New York: Cambridge University Press.

Blieszner, Rosemary. 1986. "Trends in Family Gerontology Research." *Family Relations* 35:555–562.

Blieszner, Rosemary, and Jay A. Mancini. 1987. "Enduring Ties: Older Adults' Parental Role and Responsibilities." *Family Relations* 36:176–180.

Booth, Alan, and John N. Edwards. 1992. "Starting Over: Why Remarriages Are More Unstable." *Journal of Family Issues* 13:179–194.

Borjas, George J. 1994. "The Economics of Immigration." *Journal of Economic Literature* 32:1667–1717.

Bound, John, Michael Schoenbaum, and Timothy Waidmann. 1996. "Race Differences in Labor Force Attachment and Disability Status." *The Gerontologist* 36:311–321.

Bumpass, Larry L., and James A. Sweet. 1997. National Survey of Families and House-holds: Wave 1, 1987–1988, and Wave 2, 1992–1994 [computer file]. ICPSR version. Madison: University of Wisconsin, Center for Demography and Ecology. Ann Arbor, MI: Inter-university Consortium for Political and Social Research.

Burawoy, Michael. 2000. "Marxism After Communism." *Theory and Society* 29:151–174.

Burman, Leonard E., and William G. Gale. 2001. "A Golden Opportunity to Simplify the Tax System." Brookings Policy Brief No. 77. April. Washington, DC: Brookings Institution.

Burton, Linda M., and Peggye Dilworth-Anderson. 1991. "The Intergenerational Family Roles of Aged Black Americans." *Marriage and Family Review* 15:311–330.

Burton, Lynda, Judith Kasper, Andrew Shore, Kathleen Cagney, Thomas Laveist, Catherine Cubbin, and Pearl German. 1995. "The Structure of Informal Care: Are There Differences by Race?" *The Gerontologist* 35:744–752.

Burwell, Brian O., and William H. Crown. 1994. *Public Financing of Long-Term Care: Federal and State Roles.* Washington, DC: U.S. Department of Health and Human Services.

Burwell, Brian, Mary Harahan, John Drabek, David Kennell, and Lisa Alecxih. 1993. *An Analysis of Long-Term Care Reform Proposals.* Washington, DC: U.S. Department of Health and Human Services. Retrieved August 16, 2005, from aspe.hhs.gov/daltcp/reports/REFORMES.HTM.

Calasanti, Toni, and Alessandro Bonanno. 1986. "The Social Creation of Dependence, Dependency Ratios, and the Elderly in the United States: A Critical Analysis." *Social Science and Medicine* 23:1229–1236.

Caldwell, John C. 1976. "Toward a Restatement of Demographic Transition Theory." *Population and Development Review* 2 (September–December): 321–366.

Carasso, Adam, and C. Eugene Steuerle. 2003. *The Life (and Death?) of the Estate and Gift Tax.* Washington, DC: Urban Institute.

Carelli, Richard (Associated Press). 1995. "Chief Justice's Will an Example of How Not to Handle an Estate." *The (Cleveland) Plain Dealer*, November 1.

Carreiro, Rich, Art Kamlet, and John Fisher. 2004. *Tax Code: Estate and Gift Tax.* Retrieved April 22, 2007, from invest-faq.com/articles/tax-estate-gift.html.

Casper, Lynne M., and Ken R. Bryson. 1998. *Co-Resident Grandparents and Their Grand-children: Grandparent-Maintained Families.* Census Bureau, Fertility and Family Statistics Branch. Population Division Working Paper No. 26. from www.census.gov/population/www/documentation/twps0026/twps0026.html.

Centers for Medicare and Medicaid Services. 2006. *National Health Expenditure (NHE) Amounts by Type of Expenditure and Source of Funds: Calendar Years 1965–2015.* Baltimore, MD: Centers for Medicare and Medicaid Services.

Chatters, Linda M., Robert J. Taylor, and Jason S. Jackson. 1986. "Aged Blacks' Choices for an Informal Helper Network." *Journal of Gerontology* 41:94–100.

Cherlin, Andrew. 1978. "Remarriage as an Incomplete Institution." *American Journal of Sociology* 84:634–640.

Cherlin, Andrew J., and Frank F. Furstenberg, Jr. 1994. "Stepfamilies in the United States: A Reconsideration." *Annual Review of Sociology* 20:359–382.

Choudhury, Sharmila. 2001–2002. "Racial and Ethnic Differences in Wealth and Asset Choices." *Social Security Bulletin* 64:1–15.

Clark, Margaret, and Barbara G. Anderson. 1967. *Culture and Aging: An Anthropological Study of Older Americans.* Springfield, IL: Charles C. Thomas Publisher.

Cochran, Thomas C. 1985. *Challenges to American Values: Society, Business, and Religion.* New York: Oxford University Press.

Coleman, Marilyn, Lawrence Ganong, and Susan M. Cable. 1997. "Beliefs about Women's Intergenerational Family Obligations to Provide Support Before and After Divorce and Remarriage." *Journal of Marriage and the Family* 59:165–176.

Congressional Budget Office. 2000. "Federal Spending on the Elderly and Children." Congressional Budget Office web site. Retrieved January 3, 2005, from www.cbo.gov/showdoc.cfm?index=2300&sequence=0&from=7.

Conley, Dalton. 2001. "Decomposing the Black-White Wealth Gap: The Role of Parental Resources, Inheritance, and Investment Dynamics." *Sociological Inquiry* 71:39–66.

Cooney, Teresa M., and Peter Uhlenberg. 1992. "Support from Parents over the Life Course: The Adult Child's Perspective." *Social Forces* 71:63–84.

Coughlin, Theresa A., Leighton Ku, and John Holahan. 1994. *Medicaid since 1980: Costs, Coverage, and the Shifting Alliance between the Federal Government and the States.* Washington, DC: Urban Institute.

Cox, Donald. 1987. "Motives for Private Income Transfers." *Journal of Political Economy* 95:1045–1076.

———. 2003. "Private Transfers within the Family: Mothers, Fathers, Sons, and Daughters." Pp. 168–201 in *Death and Dollars*, edited by Alicia H. Munnell and Annika Sundén. Washington, DC: Brookings Institution.

Crimmins, Eileen M., Mark D. Hayward, and Yasuhiko Saito. 1996. "Differentials in Active Life Expectancy in the Older Population of the United States." *Journals of Gerontology, Series B: Psychological Sciences and Social Sciences* 51: S111–S120.

Crimmins, Eileen M., and Dominique G. Ingegneri. 1990. "Interaction and Living Arrangements of Older Parents and Their Children: Past Trends, Present Determinants, Future Implications." *Research on Aging* 12:3–35.

Cronin, Julie-Anne. 1999. "U.S. Treasury Distributional Analysis Methodology." Office of Tax Analysis Paper No. 85. Washington, DC: U.S. Department of the Treasury.

Crystal, Stephen. 1984. *America's Old-Age Crisis: Public Policy and the Two Worlds of Aging.* New York: Basic Books.

Crystal, Stephen, and Dennis Shea. 1990. "The Economic Well-being of the Elderly." *Review of Income and Wealth* 36:227–247.

———. 2003. "Cumulative Advantage, Public Policy, and Inequality in Later Life." *Annual Review of Gerontology and Geriatrics* 22:1–13.

Crystal, Stephen, Dennis Shea, and Shereeram Krishnaswami. 1992. "Educational Attainment, Occupational History, and Stratification: Determinants of Later-life Economic Outcomes." *Journal of Gerontology: Social Sciences* 47: S213–S221.

Curran, Barbara A. 1989. *Report on the 1989 Survey of the Public's Use of Legal Services.* Washington, DC: American Bar Association Consortium on Legal Services and the Public, and Tulane Law School.

Dang, Thai-Thanh, Pablo Antolin, and Howard Oxley. 2001. "Fiscal Implications of Ageing: Projections of Age-related Spending." Retrieved July 7, 2004, from www.nabe.com/ps2000/jamesohd.pdf.

Davis, Kingsley, and Pietronella van den Oever. 1981. "Age Relations and Public Policy in Advanced Industrial Societies." *Population and Development Review* 7:1–18.

Deflem, Mathieu. 2003. "The Sociology of the Sociology of Money: Simmel and the Contemporary Battle of the Classics." *Journal of Classical Sociology* 3:67–96.

Degler, Carl. 1980. *At Odds: Women and the Family in America from the Revolution to the Present.* New York: Oxford University Press.

DeNavas-Walt, Carmen, Bernadette D. Proctor, and Cheryl Hill Lee. 2006. *Income, Poverty, and Health Insurance Coverage in the United States: 2005.* Current Population Survey P60-231. Washington, DC: Government Printing Office.

Derthick, Martha, and Steven M. Teles. 2003. "Riding the Third Rail: Social Security Reform." Pp. 182–208 in *The Reagan Presidency: Pragmatic Conservatism and Its Legacies,* edited by W. Elliot Brownlee and Hugh Davis. Lawrence: University Press of Kansas.

De Vos, Susan, and Elizabeth Arias. 2001. *A First Look at Living Arrangements among Hispanic Elders, 1970–2000, with Special Emphasis on Living Alone among Unmarried Women.* Center for Demography and Ecology Working Paper No. 2001-5. Madison: University of Wisconsin.

Dietz, Tracy L. 1995. "Patterns of Intergenerational Assistance within the Mexican-American Family." *Journal of Family Issues* 16:344–356.

Dilworth-Anderson, Peggye. 1992. "Extended Kin Networks in Black Families." *Generations* 16:29–32.

Douglas, Mary. 1990. "Foreword: No Free Gifts." Pp. vii–xviii in *The Gift: The Form and Reason for Exchange in Archaic Societies,* by M. Mauss. New York: W. W. Norton.

Dukeminier, Jesse, and Stanley M. Johanson. 2000. *Wills, Trusts and Estates,* 6th edition. Gaithersburg, MD: Aspen Law and Business Publishing.

Dunn, Thomas A., and John W. Phillips. 1997. "The Timing and Division of Parental Transfers to Children." *Economics Letters* 54:135–138.

Eggebeen, David J. 1992. "Family Structure and Intergenerational Exchanges." *Research on Aging* 14:427–447.

Eisenberg, Howard B. 1991. "Durable Power of Attorney v. Living Will: Counseling Older Clients." *Illinois Bar Journal* 79:384–389.

Elo, I. T., and S. H. Preston. 1997. "Racial and Ethnic Differences in American Mortality at Older Ages." Pp. 10–42 in *Racial and Ethnic Differences in the Health of Older Ameri-*

cans, edited by Linda Martin and Beth Soldo. Washington, DC: National Academy Press.

Emerson, Richard. 1962. "Power-Dependence Relations." *American Sociological Review* 27:31–41.

Esping-Andersen, Gøsta. 1990. *The Three Worlds of Welfare Capitalism*. Princeton, NJ: Princeton University Press.

———. 1996. *Welfare States in Transition: Social Security in the New Global Economy*. London: Sage.

———. 1999. *The Social Foundations of Postindustrial Economies*. Oxford: Oxford University Press.

———. 2002. *Why We Need a New Welfare State*. Oxford: Oxford University Press.

Estes, Carroll. 1979. *Aging Enterprise: A Critical Examination of Social Policies and Services for the Aged*. San Francisco: Jossey-Bass.

Estes, Carroll L., and Associates. 2001. *Social Policy and Aging: A Critical Perspective*. Thousand Oaks, CA: Sage Publications.

Etzioni, Amitai. 1988. *The Moral Dimension: Toward a New Economics*. New York: Free Press.

Farrell, H. Clyde. 2001. *Financing Long-Term Care in Texas*, edition 7.1. Austin, TX.

Finch, Janet, and Lynn Hayes. 1994. "Inheritance, Death, and the Concept of the Home." *Sociology* 28:417–433.

Fish, Barry, and Les Kotzer. 2002. *The Family Fight: Planning to Avoid It*. Thornhill, Ontario: Continental Atlantic Publications.

Fredman, Lisa, Mel P. Daly, and Ann M. Lazur. 1995. "Burden among White and Black Caregivers to Elderly Adults." *Journal of Gerontology* 50B: S110–S118.

Freedman, Vicki A., Douglas A. Wolf, Beth J. Soldo, and Elizabeth H. Stephen. 1991. "Intergenerational Transfers: A Question of Perspective." *The Gerontologist* 31:640–647.

Galbraith, Jamie, and Maureen Berner, eds. 2001. *Inequality and Industrial Change: A Global View*. New York: Cambridge University Press.

Gale, William G., and John K. Scholz. 1994. "Intergenerational Transfers and the Accumulation of Wealth." *Journal of Economic Perspectives* 8:145–160.

Gates, William H., Sr., and Chuck Collins. 2003. "A Fair Payment for War." *Washington Post*. March 25. Retrieved July 7, 2004, from www.responsiblewealth.org/press/rwnews/2003/Gates_Collins_Wash_Post_Op.html.

General Accounting Office. 1989. *Medicaid: Recoveries from Nursing Home Residents' Estates Could Offset Program Costs*. GAO/HRD-89-56. Washington, DC: Government Printing Office.

———. 1996. *401(k) Pension Plans. Many Take Advantage of Opportunity to Ensure Adequate Retirement Income*. GAO/HEHS-96-176. Washington, DC: Government Printing Office.

———. 2002. "Long-Term Care: Aging Baby Boom Generation Will Increase Demand and Burden on Federal and State Budgets." Testimony by David M. Walker, Comptroller General of the United States, before the Senate Special Committee on Aging. GAO-02-544T. Washington, DC: Government Printing Office.

Georgetown University Long-Term Care Financing Project. 2007. *Fact Sheet: National*

Spending for Long-Term Care. Washington, DC: Health Policy Institute, Georgetown University.

Gibson, Rose C. 1986. "Older Black Americans." *Generations* (Summer): 35–39.

Gist, John. 2006. *Boomers in Their Dreams: What Will Boomers Inherit?* Washington, DC: AARP Public Policy Institute. Available at www.aarp.org/research/reference/boomers/dd139_inherit.html.

Gist, John, and Carlos Figueiredo. 2006. "In Their Dreams: What Will Boomers Inherit?" Research Report. Washington, DC: AARP Public Policy Institute.

Glater, Jonathan D., and Alan Finder. 2006. "In New Twist on Tuition Game, Popularity Rises with the Price." *New York Times*. December 12, A1, A28.

Gokhale, Jagadeesh, and Laurence J. Kotlikoff. 2000. *The Baby Boomers' Mega-Inheritance: Myth or Reality? Economic Commentary*. Federal Reserve Bank of Cleveland. From people.bu.edu./kotlikoff/1001.pdf.

Goldscheider, Frances K., and Calvin Goldscheider. 1989. "The New Family Economy: Residential and Economic Relationships among the Generations." Pp. 1–16 in *Ethnicity and the New Family Economy: Living Arrangements and Intergenerational Financial Flows*, edited by Frances K. Goldscheider and Calvin Goldscheider. Boulder, CO: Westview.

———. 1991. "The Intergenerational Flow of Income: Family Structure and the Status of Black Americans." *Journal of Marriage and the Family* 53:499–508.

Graeber, David. 2001. *Toward an Anthropological Theory of Value*. New York: Palgrave.

Greenberg, Jan S., and Marion Becker. 1988. "Aging Parents as Family Resources." *The Gerontologist* 28:786–791.

Greene, Kelly. 2002. "Money Matters: Pass It On." *Wall Street Journal*, March 25, R5.

Groger, Lisa. 1992. "Tied to Each Other through Ties to the Land: Informal Support of Black Elders in a Southern U.S. Community." *Journal of Cross-Cultural Gerontology* 7:205–220.

Groger, Lisa, and Suzanne Kunkel. 1995. "Aging and Exchange: Differences between Black and White Elders." *Journal of Cross-Cultural Gerontology* 10:269–287.

Gross, Jane. 2006. "Elder-Care Costs Deplete Savings of a Generation." *New York Times*. December 30, A1, A16.

Gruber, Jonathan. 2003. "Bequest: By Accident or by Design? Comments." Pp. 126–129 in *Death and Dollars*, edited by Alicia H. Munnell and Annika Sundén. Washington, DC: Brookings Institution.

Gruber, Jonathan, and Brigitte C. Madrian. 1995. "Health Insurance Availability and the Retirement Decision." *American Economic Review* 85:938–948.

Grundy, Emily. 2005. "Reciprocity in Relationships: Socio-economic and Health Influences on Intergenerational Exchanges between Third Age Parents and Their Adult Children in Great Britain." *British Journal of Sociology* 56:233–255.

Gustman, Alan L., and Thomas L. Steinmeier. 2003. "What People Don't Know about Their Pensions and Social Security: An Analysis Using Linked Data from the Health and Retirement Study." Pp. 57–125 in *Public Policies and Private Pensions*, edited by William G. Gale, John B. Shoven, and Mark J. Warshawsky. Washington, DC: Brookings Institution.

Haider, Steven J., Alison Jacknowitz, and Robert F. Schoeni. 2003. "The Economic Status of Elderly Divorced Women." Retrieved January 3, 2005, from www.mrrc.isr.umich .edu/research/publications/Conference_Paper/HaiderShoeni_0208.pdf.

Hall, Peter D., and George E. Marcus. 1998. "Why Should Men Leave Great Fortunes to Their Children? Class, Dynasty, and Inheritance in America." Pp. 139–171 in *Inheritance and Wealth in America*, edited by R. K. Miller and S. J. McNamee. New York: Plenum Press.

Hanson, Sandra L., William J. Sauer, and Wayne C. Seelbach. 1983. "Racial and Cohort Variations in Filial Responsibility Norms." *The Gerontologist* 23:626–631.

Hareven, Tamara K. 1977. *Introduction to Family and Kin in Urban Communities, 1700–1930.* New York: New Viewpoints.

Harrington, Charlene, Christine Cassel, Carroll L. Estes, Steffie Woolhandler, and David U. Himmelstein. 1991. "A National Long-term Care Program for the United States." *Journal of the American Medical Association* 266:3023–3029.

Harris, Gardiner. 2005. "Gee, Fixing Welfare Seemed Like a Snap." *New York Times.* June 19, section 4, p. 3.

Hashimoto, Akiko. 1996. *The Gift of Generations: Japanese and American Perspectives on Aging and the Social Contract.* New York: Cambridge University Press.

Havens, John J., and Paul G. Schervish. 1999. "Millionaires and the Millennium: New Estimates of the Forthcoming Wealth Transfer and the Prospects for a Golden Age of Philanthropy." Social Welfare Policy Research Institute Report. Chestnut Hill, MA: Boston College Center on Wealth and Philanthropy. Retrieved July 7, 2004, from www.bc.edu/bc_org/avp/gsas/SWPI/documents/m&m.pdf.

———. 2002. *The Identification Theory and the Allocation of Transfers between Family and Philanthropic Organizations.* Chestnut Hill, MA: Boston College Social Welfare Research Institute.

———. 2003a. "Why the $41 Trillion Wealth Transfer Is Still Valid: A Review of Challenges and Questions." *Journal of Gift Planning* 7: 11–15, 47–50.

———. 2003b. "Millionaires and the Millennium: New Estimates of the Forthcoming Wealth Transfer and the Prospects for a Golden Age of Philanthropy." Social Welfare Policy Research Institute Report. Chestnut Hill, MA: Boston College Center on Wealth and Philanthropy. Retrieved July 7, 2004, from www.bc.edu/research/swri/meta-eleme nts/pdf/m_m.pdf.

Heffler, Stephen, Sheila Smith, Sean Keehan, M. Kent Clemens, Greg Won, and Mark Zezza. 2003. "Health Spending Projections for 2002–2012." *Health Affairs* 22:W3-54–W3-65. Retrieved August 4, 2004, from content.healthaffairs.org/cgi/content/abstract/ hlthaff.w3.54.

Hendlin, Steven J. 2004. *Overcoming the Inheritance Taboo.* New York: Penguin.

Hendricks, Jon, Laurie Russell, and Stephen J. Cutler. 1999. "Entitlements, Social Compacts, and the Trend toward Retrenchment in U.S. Old-Age Programs." *Hallym International Journal of Aging* 1:14–32.

Henretta, James A. 1973. *The Evolution of American Society, 1780–1815.* Lexington, MA: D. C. Heath.

Henretta John C., Emily Grundy, and Susan Harris. 2001. "Socio-economic Differences in Having Living Parents and Children: A US-British Comparison of Middle-aged Women." *Journal of Marriage and Family* 63:852–867.

———. 2002. "The Influence of Socio-economic and Health Differences on Parents' Provision of Help to Adult Children: A British–United States Comparison." *Ageing and Society* 22:441–458.

Henretta, John C., Martha S. Hill, Wei Li, Beth J. Soldo, and Douglas A. Wolf. 1997. "Selection of Children to Provide Care: The Effect of Earlier Parental Transfers." *Journal of Gerontology: Social Sciences* 52B (special issue): 110–119.

Herd, Pamela. 2005. "Ensuring a Minimum: Social Security Reform and Women." *The Gerontologist* 45:12–25.

———. 2006. "Crediting Care or Marriage? Reforming Social Security Family Benefits." *Journal of Gerontology: Social Sciences* 61B: S24–S34.

Hess, Beth B., and Joan M. Waring. 1978. "Parent and Child in Later Life: Rethinking the Relationship." Pp. 241–273 in *Child Influences on Marital and Family Interaction*, edited by Richard M. Lerner and Graham B. Spanier. New York: Academic Press.

Hill, Martha S. 1992. "The Role of Economic Resources and Remarriage in Financial Assistance for Children of Divorce." *Journal of Family Issues* 13:158–178.

Himes, Christine L., Dennis P. Hogan, and David J. Eggebeen. 1996. "Living Arrangements of Minority Elders." *Journal of Gerontology* 51B: S42–S48.

Hochgraf, Eva S. 1999. "Sermon based on the book *The Gift: Imagination and the Erotic Life of Property*." Retrieved July 8, 2004, from www.uuaa.org/sermons/thegift.txt.

Hoffer, Peter Charles. 1992. *Law and People in Colonial America*. Baltimore: Johns Hopkins University Press.

Hogan, Dennis P., and David J. Eggebeen. 1995. "Sources of Emergency Help and Routine Assistance in Old Age." *Social Forces* 73:917–936.

Hogan, Dennis P., David J. Eggebeen, and Clifford C. Clogg. 1993. "The Structure of Intergenerational Exchanges in American Families." *American Journal of Sociology* 98:1428–1458.

Hogan, Dennis P., Ling-Xin Hao, and William L. Parish. 1990. "Race, Kin Networks, and Assistance to Mother-Headed Families." *Social Forces* 68:797–812.

Holahan, John, and John L. Palmer. 1988. "Medicare's Fiscal Problems: An Imperative for Reform." *Journal of Health Politics, Policy, and Law* 13:53–81.

Holden, Karen, and Daphne Kuo. 1996. "Complex Marital Histories and Economic Wellbeing: The Continuing Legacy of Divorce and Widowhood as the HRS Cohort Approaches Retirement." *The Gerontologist* 36:383–390.

Holden, Karen C., and Timothy M. Smeeding. 1990. "The Poor, the Rich, and the Insecure Caught in Between." *Milbank Quarterly* 68:191–219.

Holden, Karen C., and Pamela J. Smock. 1991. "The Economic Costs of Marital Dissolution: Why Do Women Bear a Disproportionate Cost?" *Annual Review of Sociology* 17:51–78.

Hollmann, Frederick W., Tammany J. Mulder, and Jeffrey E. Kallan. 2000. "Methodology and Assumptions for the Population Projections of the United States, 1999 to 2100." Population Division Working Paper No. 38. Washington, DC: U.S. Census Bureau. Retrieved July 18, 2004, from www.census.gov/population/documentation/twps0038/tabC.txt.

Holzmann, Robert, and Joseph E. Stiglitz, eds. 2001. *New Ideas about Old Age Security: Toward Sustainable Pension Systems in the Twenty-First Century.* Washington, DC: World Bank.

Homans, George C. 1958. "Social Behavior as Exchange." *American Journal of Sociology* 63:597–606.

———. 1974. *Social Behavior: Its Elementary Forms,* 2nd edition. New York: Harcourt Brace Jovanovich.

Honig, Majorie. 2000. "Minorities Face Retirement: Worklife Disparities Repeated?" Pp. 235–252 in *Forecasting Retirement Needs and Retirement Wealth,* edited by B. Hammond, O. S. Mitchell, and A. Rappaport. Philadelphia: University of Pennsylvania Press.

Hoyert, Donna L., Kenneth D. Kochanek, and Sherry L. Murphy. 1999. "Deaths: Final Data for 1997." *National Vital Statistics Report* 47:1–105.

Hubbard, R. Glenn, Jonathan Skinner, and Stephen P. Zeldes. 1995. "Precautionary Saving and Social Insurance." *Journal of Political Economy* 103:360–399.

Hudson, Robert B. 1978. "The 'Graying' of the Federal Budget and Its Consequences for Old-Age Policy." *The Gerontologist* 14:428–440.

———. 1999. "Conflict in Aging Politics: New Population Encounters Old Ideology." *Social Service Review* 73:358–379.

———, ed. 2005. *The New Politics of Old Age Policy.* Baltimore: Johns Hopkins University Press.

Hughes, M. Elizabeth, and Angela M. O'Rand. 2004. *The Lives and Times of the Baby Boomers.* New York: Russell Sage Foundation.

Hurd, Michael D. 2003. "Bequests: By Accident or by Design?" Pp. 93–118 in *Death and Dollars,* edited by A. H. Munnell and A. Sundén. Washington, DC: Brookings Institution.

Hurd, Michael D., and James P. Smith. 2002. "Expected Bequests and Their Distributions." Working Paper 9142. Cambridge, MA: National Bureau of Economic Research. Retrieved July 7, 2004, from www.nber.org/papers/W9142.

Hyde, Lewis. 1983. *The Gift: Imagination and the Erotic Life of Property.* New York: Vintage.

Institute of Medicine. 2004. *Insuring America's Health: Principles and Recommendations.* Washington, DC: National Academy Press.

Internal Revenue Service. 2006. Table 5c. In *Estate Tax Returns Filed in 2000: Gross Estate, Total Deductions, State Death Tax Credits, and Estate Tax After Credits, by State of Residence.* Available at www.irs.gov/pub/irs-soi/00es05c.xls.

James, Estelle. 1994. *Averting the Old Age Crisis: Policies to Protect the Old and Promote Growth.* Washington, DC: Oxford University Press and The World Bank.

———. 2001. "Reforming Social Security in the U.S.: An International Perspective." *Journal of Business Economics* (January): 16–31.

Jamieson, Amie, Hyon B. Shin, and Jennifer Day. 2002. "Voting and Registration in the Election of November 2000." *Current Population Reports* (February): P20-542. Washington, DC: U.S. Census Bureau.

Jayakody, Rukmalie. 1998. "Race Differences in Intergenerational Financial Assistance:

The Needs of Children and the Resources of Parents." *Journal of Family Issues* 19 (5): 508–533.

Johnson, Richard W., and Melissa Favreault. 2004. *Economic Status in Later Life among Women Who Raised Children Outside of Marriage*. Washington, DC: Urban Institute.

Johnson, Richard W., Usha Sambamoorthi, and Stephen Crystal. 2003. "Gender Differences in Pension Wealth and Their Impact on Late-life Inequality." Pp. 116–137 in *Annual Review of Gerontology and Geriatrics*, edited by S. Crystal and D. Shea. New York: Springer.

Juster, F. Thomas, and Richard Suzman. 1995. "The Health and Retirement Study: An Overview." *Journal of Human Resources* 30 (supplement): S7–S56.

Kahn, Robert C., and Toni C. Antonucci. 1981. *Convoys of Social Support: A Life-course Approach*. Pp. 383–405 in *Aging: Social Change*, edited by Sara B. Kiesler and Valerie K. Oppenheimer. New York: Academic Press.

Kane, Thomas J., and Peter R. Orszag. 2003. "Funding Restrictions at Public Universities: Effects and Policy Implications." Brookings Institution Tax Policy Center Working Paper No. 124. Washington, DC: Brookings Institution.

Katz, Stanley N. 1977–1978. "Republicanism and the Law of Inheritance in the American Revolutionary Era." *Michigan Law Review* 76:1–29.

Kennickell, Arthur B., Martha Starr-McCluer, and Annika E. Sundén. 1996. *Saving and Financial Planning: Some Findings from a Focus Group*. Washington, DC: Federal Reserve Board of Governors.

Kingson, Eric R. 1986. "Intergenerational Inequity: Why It Won't Work as a Framework for Policy." Pp. 129–159 in *Ties That Bind*, by Eric R. Kingson, Barbara A. Hirshorn, and John M. Cornman. Cabin John, MD: Seven Locks Press.

Kingson, Eric R., and Edward D. Berkowitz. 1994. "Social Security: Will Successive Generations Receive Fair Returns." *Perspectives on Aging* 23:15–18.

Kingson, Eric R., Barbara A. Hirshorn, and John M. Cornman. 1986. *Ties That Bind: The Interdependence of Generations*, Cabin John, MD: Seven Locks Press.

Kingson, Eric R., and Uwe Reinhardt, eds. 2000. *Social Security and Medicare: Individual vs. Collective Crisis and Responsibilities*. Washington, DC: Brookings Institution and National Academy of Social Insurance.

Kingson, Eric R., and James H. Schulz, eds. 1997. *Social Security in the 21st Century*. New York: Oxford University Press.

Kopczuk, Wojciech, and Joel Slemrod. 2003. "Tax Consequences on Wealth Accumulation and Transfers of the Rich." Pp. 213–264 in *Death and Dollars*, edited by A. H. Munnell and A. Sundén. Washington, DC: Brookings Institution.

Kotlikoff, Laurence J., and Scott Burns. 2005. *The Coming Generational Storm. What You Need to Know*. Cambridge: MIT Press.

Kotlikoff, Laurence J., and Lawrence H. Summers. 1981. "The Role of Intergenerational Transfers in Aggregate Capital Accumulation." *Journal of Political Economy* 89:706–732.

Krueger, Richard A. 1994. *Focus Groups: A Practical Guide for Applied Research*, 2nd ed. Thousand Oaks, CA: Sage Publications.

Lamm, Richard D. 2003. *The Brave New World of Health Care*. Golden, CO: Fulcrum Publishing.

Langbein, John H. 1988. "The Twentieth-Century Revolution in Family Wealth Transmission." *Michigan Law Review* 86:722–751.

Langbein, John H., and Bruce A. Wolk. 2004. *Pension and Employee Benefit Law*. New York: Foundation Press.

Laslett, Peter. 1987. "The Character of Familial History, Its Limitations and the Conditions for Its Proper Pursuit." *Journal of Family History* 12:263–284.

———. 1991. *Fresh Map of Life: The Emergence of the Third Age*. Cambridge: Harvard University Press.

Lawrence, Renee H., Joan M. Bennett, and Kyriakos S. Markides. 1992. "Perceived Intergenerational Solidarity and Psychological Distress among Older Mexican Americans." *Journal of Gerontology: Social Sciences* 47:55–65.

Lawton, Leora, Merril Silverstein, and Vern L. Bengtson. 1994. "Solidarity between Generations in Families." Pp. 19–42 in *Intergenerational Linkages: Hidden Connections in American Society*. New York: Springer.

Lee, Gary R., and Eugene Ellithorpe. 1982. "Intergenerational Exchange and Subjective Well-Being among the Elderly." *Journal of Marriage and the Family* 44:217–224.

Lee, Yean-Ju, and Isik A. Aytac. 1998. "Intergenerational Financial Support among Whites, African-Americans, and Latinos." *Journal of Marriage and the Family* 60:426–441.

Lévi-Strauss, Claude. 1969. *The Elementary Structures of Kinship*. London: Eyre and Spottiswoode.

Levitt, Mary J., Nathalie Guacci, and Ruth A. Weber. 1992. "Intergenerational Support, Relationship Quality, and Well-Being: A Bicultural Analysis." *Journal of Family Issues* 13:465–481.

Lewin, Tamara. 2005. "Financially Set Grandparents Help Keep Families Afloat, Too." *New York Times*, July 14, A1, A22.

Libecap, Gary D., and Zeynep K. Hansen. 2001. "U.S. Land Policy, Property Rights, and the Dust Bowl of the 1930s." FEEM Working Paper No. 69.2001. Available at ssrn.com/abstract=286699 or 10.2139/ssrn.286699.

Lin, Ge, and Peter A. Rogerson. 1995. "Elderly Parents and the Geographic Availability of Their Adult Children." *Research on Aging* 17:303–331.

Lown, Jean M., Joan R. McFadden, and Sharyn M. Crossman. 1989. "Family Life Education for Remarriage: Focus on Financial Management." *Family Relations* 38:40–45.

Lye, Diana N. 1996. "Adult Child-Parent Relationships." *Annual Review of Sociology* 22: 79–102.

Lye, Diana N., Daniel H. Kleplinger, Patricia Davis Hyle, and Anjanette Nelson. 1995. "Childhood Living Arrangements and Adult Children's Relations with Their Parents." *Demography* 32:261–280.

Maclachlan, Fiona. 2003. *Interest, an Historical and Analytical Study in Economics and Modern Ethics*. Milwaukee, WI: Marquette University Press.

Mancini, Jay A., and Rosemary Blieszner. 1989. "Aging Parents and Adult Children: Research Themes in Intergenerational Relations." *Journal of Marriage and the Family* 51:275–290.

Markides, Kyriakos S., Joanne S. Boldt, and Laura A. Ray. 1986. "Sources of Helping and Intergenerational Solidarity: A Three-Generations Study of Mexican Americans." *Journal of Gerontology: Social Sciences* 41:506–551.

Markides, Kyriakos S., Harry W. Martin, and Ernesto Gomez. 1983. "Older Mexican Americans: A Study in an Urban Barrio." Austin: University of Texas.

Mastracco, Anna. 1994. "Federal and State Coordination: Medicaid-State Plans and Financing." *Administrative Law Review* 46:481–510.

Mauss, Marcel. 1990. *The Gift: The Form and Reason for Exchange in Archaic Societies.* London: Routledge.

Mayer, J. P., ed. 1969. *Democracy in America: Alexis de Tocqueville.* Garden City, NY: Anchor Books.

McAdoo, Harriette Pipes. 1978. "Factors Related to Stability in Upwardly Mobile Black Families." *Journal of Marriage and the Family* 40:761–776.

McClellan, David. 1979. *Marxism after Marx.* New York: Houghton Mifflin.

McGarry, Kathleen, and Robert F. Schoeni. 1995. "Transfer Behavior in the Health and Retirement Study: Measurement and the Redistribution of Resources within the Family." *Journal of Human Resources* 30: S184–S226.

———. 1997. "Transfer Behavior within the Family: Results for the Asset and Health Dynamics Study." *Journal of Gerontology: Social Sciences* 52B (special issue): 82–92.

McLanahan, Sara, and Gary Sandefur. 1994. *Growing Up with a Single Parent: What Hurts? What Helps?* Cambridge: Harvard University Press.

Menchik, Paul L., and Nancy Ammon Jianakoplos. 1997. "Black-White Wealth Inequality: Is Inheritance the Reason?" *Economic Inquiry* 35:428–442.

MetLife. 2002. "Who Pays for Long-term Care?" Retrieved November 30, 2006, from www.metlife.com/Applications/Corporate/WPS/CDA/PageGenerator/0,4132,P1863 ,00.html.

Miller, Robert K., Jr., and Stephen J. McNamee, eds. 1998. *Inheritance and Wealth in America.* New York: Plenum Press.

Mindel, Charles H., Roosevelt Wright, Jr., and R. A. Starrett. 1986. "Informal and Formal Health and Social Support Systems of Black and White Elderly: Comparative Cost Approach." *The Gerontologist* 26:279–285.

Miner, Sonia. 1995. "Racial Differences in Family Support and Formal Service Utilization among Older Persons: A Non-Recursive Model." *Journal of Gerontology* 50B: S143–S153.

Minkler, Meredith, and Kathleen Roe. 1993. *Grandmothers as Caregivers: Raising Children of the Crack Cocaine Epidemic.* Newbury Park, CA: Sage.

Minkler, Meredith, Kathleen Roe, and Marilyn Price. 1992. "The Physical and Emotional Health of Grandmothers Raising Grandchildren in the Crack Cocaine Epidemic." *The Gerontologist* 32:752–760.

Mitchell, Daniel J. B. 2000. *Pensions, Politics, and the Elderly: Historic Social Movements and Their Lessons for Our Aging Society.* Armonk, NY: M. E. Sharpe.

Mitchell, J., and J. C. Register. 1984. "An Exploration of Family Interaction with the Elderly by Race, Socioeconomic Status, and Residence." *The Gerontologist* 24:48–54.

Mitchell, Olivia S., and James F. Moore. 1998. "Can Americans Afford to Retire? New Evidence on Retirement Saving Adequacy." *Journal of Risk and Insurance* 65:371–400.

Molm, Linda D., and Karen S. Cook. 1995. "Social Exchange and Exchange Networks." Pp. 209–235 in *Sociological Perspectives on Social Psychology*, edited by Karen S. Cook, Gary Alan Fine, and James S. House. Boston: Allyn and Bacon.

Moon, Marilyn. 2000. *Competition with Constraints: Challenges Facing Medicare Reform.* Washington, DC: Urban Institute.

Morgan, Leslie A. 1983. "Intergenerational Financial Support: Retirement-Age Males, 1971–1975." *The Gerontologist* 23:160–166.

Mui, Ada C. 1992. "Caregiver Strain among Black and White Daughter Caregivers: A Role Theory Perspective." *The Gerontologist* 32:203–212.

Munnell, Alicia H. 2003. "Introduction." Pp. 1–29 in *Death and Dollars*, edited by A. H. Munnell and A. Sundén. Washington, DC: Brookings Institution.

Munnell, Alicia H., and Annika Sundén, eds. 2003. *Death and Dollars*. Washington, DC: Brookings Institution.

Munnell, Alicia, Annika Sundén, Mauricio Soto, and Catherine Taylor. 2003. "The Impact of Defined Contribution Plans on Bequests." Pp. 265–306 in *Death and Dollars*, edited by Alicia H. Munnell and Annika Sundén. Washington, DC: Brookings Institution.

Myles, John. 2002. *Why We Need a New Welfare State*. New York: Oxford University Press.

Narrett, David E. 1992. *Inheritance and Family Life in Colonial New York City*. Ithaca, NY: Cornell University Press.

Neikirk, William. 2005. "Social Security Fight Begins." *Sun Journal*. www.snowe.senate .gov/articles/art042705_1.htm.

Ng-Baumhackl, Mitja, John Gist, and Carlos Figueiredo. 2003. "Pennies from Heaven: Will Inheritances Bail Out the Boomers?" Washington, DC: AARP Public Policy Institute.

O'Brien, Ellen. 2005. *Long-Term Care: Understanding Medicaid's Role for the Elderly and Disabled*. Washington, DC: Kaiser Commission on Medicaid and the Uninsured.

O'Brien, Ellen, and Risa Elias. 2004. *Long-term Care and Medicaid*. Washington, DC: Kaiser Commission on Medicaid and the Uninsured.

O'Connor, Colleen. 1996. "Empirical Research on How the Elderly Handle Their Estates." *Generations* 20:13–20.

Office of the Assistant Secretary for Planning and Evaluation. 2005. "Growth of Medical Expenditures—Public and Private: ASPE Issue Brief." Washington, DC. Retrieved December 15, 2006, from aspe.hhs.gov/health/medicalexpenditures.

O'Rand, Angela M. 1996. "The Precious and the Precocious: Understanding Cumulative Disadvantage and Cumulative Advantage over the Life Course." *The Gerontologist* 36:230–258.

———. 2001. "Stratification and the Life Course: The Forms of Life-Course Capital and Their Interrelationships." Pp. 197–237 in *Handbook of Aging and the Social Sciences*, edited by Robert H. Binstock and Linda K. George. San Diego: Academic Press.

Organization for Economic Co-operation and Development. 1998. *Maintaining Prosperity in an Ageing Society*. Paris: OECD Publishing.

Ostrom, Carol M. 2004. "Medical Debt Blamed for Rise in Personal Bankruptcies. *Seattle Times*, June 25. Retrieved July 6, 2004, from seattletimes.nwsource.com/html/local news/2001965063_bankruptcies25m.html.

Padavic, Irene, and Barbara Reskin. 2002. *Women and Men at Work*. Thousand Oaks, CA: Pine Forge Press.

Palloni, Alberto, Beth Soldo, and Rebeca Wong. 2002. "Health Status in a National Sample of Elderly Mexicans." Paper prepared for presentation at the Gerontological Society of America conference, Boston, November.

Palmer, John L., and Thomas R. Saving. 2004. "Status of the Social Security and Medicare Programs: A Summary of the 2004 Annual Reports." Social Security Administration, Office of the Chief Actuary. Retrieved January 3, 2005, from www.ssa.gov/OACT/TRSUM/trsummary.html.

Paz, Juan, and Sara Aleman. 1998. "The Yaqui Elderly of Old Pascua." Pp. 47–59 in *Latino Elders and the Twenty-First Century: Issues and Challenges for Culturally Competent Research and Practice*, edited by Melvin Delgado. New York: Haworth Press.

Perry, C. M., and Collen L. Johnson. 1994. "Families and Support Networks among African American Oldest-Old." *International Journal of Aging and Human Development* 38:41–50.

Pestieau, Pierre. 2003. "The Role of Gift and Estate Transfers in the United States and in Europe." Pp. 64–90 in *Death and Dollars*, edited by A. H. Munnell and A. Sundén. Washington, DC: Brookings Institution.

Peterson, Peter G. 1999. *Gray Dawn: How the Coming Age Wave Will Transform America—and the World*. New York: Times Books.

Polanyi, Karl. 1944. *The Great Transformation: The Political and Economic Origins of Our Time*. New York: Rinehart.

Prendergast, Thomas J. 2001. "Advance Care Planning: Pitfall, Progress, Promise." *Critical Care Medicine* 29 (2): 34–39.

Preston, Samuel H. 1984. "Children and the Elderly: Divergent Paths for America's Dependents." *Demography* 21:435–457.

Princeton Survey Research Associates. 1998. "Pew Research Center for the People and the Press." Retrieved July 3, 2004, from people-press.org/reports/print.php3?PageID=604.

Rafool, Mandy. 1999. *Fiscal Affairs: State Death Taxes*. National Conference of State Legislatures. Retrieved July 7, 2004, from www.Ncsl.Org/Programs/Fiscal/Deathtax.htm.

Rhodes, Robert P. 1992. *Health Care Politics, Policy, and Distributive Justice: The Ironic Triumph*. Albany: State University of New York Press. Pp. 81–93.

Ribar, David C., and Mark O. Wilhelm. 2006. "Exchange, Role Modeling and the Intergenerational Transmission of Elder Support Attitudes: Evidence from Three Generations of Mexican-Americans." *Journal of Socio-Economics* 35:514–531.

Richman, Louis S. 1994. "Who Will Inherit Your Wealth?" *Fortune* 130:125–127.

Rosenbaum, Walter A., and James W. Button. 1993. "The Unquiet Future of Intergenerational Politics." *The Gerontologist* 33:481–490.

Rosenfeld, Jeffrey P. 1979. *The Legacy of Aging: Inheritance and Disinheritance in Social Perspective*. Norwood, NJ: Ablex.

Rosenzweig, Mark R., and Kenneth I. Wolpin. 1993. "Intergenerational Support and the Life-Cycle Incomes of Young Men and Their Parents: Human Capital Investments, Coresidence, and Intergenerational Financial Transfers." *Journal of Labor Economics* 11:84–112.

Rossi, Alice, and Peter Rossi. 1990. *Of Human Bonding: Parent-Child Relations across the Life Course*. New York: Aldine de Gruyter.

Rudy, Sharon R. 1991. "Practical and Ethical Aspects of Serving Elderly Clients." *Illinois Bar Journal* 79:410–413.

———. 1996. "Substituted Decision-Making for the Elderly: Living Wills, POAs, and Other Options." *Illinois Bar Journal* 84:32–35.

Ruggles, Stephen. 1987. *Prolonged Connections: The Rise of the Extended Family in Nineteenth-Century England and America.* Madison: University of Wisconsin Press.

Salmon, Marylynn. 1986. *Women and the Law of Property in Early America.* Chapel Hill: University of North Carolina Press.

Samuelson, P. 1958. "An Exact Consumption-Loan Model of Interest With or Without the Social Contrivance of Money." *Journal of Political Economy* 66:467–482.

Schaefer, Wendy. 2000. Transcript of interview on estate planning. "Mature Texas," June 19. Travis County Television (TC-TV 17), Austin, TX.

Schervish, Paul G., and John J. Havens. 2003. "Gifts and Bequests: Family or Philanthropic Organizations?" Pp. 130–158 in *Dollars and Death*, edited by A. H. Munnell and A. Sundén. Washington, DC: Brookings Institution.

Schulz, James H., and Robert H. Binstock. 2006. *Aging Nation: The Economics and Politics of Growing Older in America.* Westport, CT: Praeger.

Schwartz, T. P. 1993. "Testamentary Behavior: Issues and Evidence about Individuality, Altruism and Social Influences." *Sociological Quarterly* 34:337–355.

———. 2000. "Disinheritance and Will Contests as Reciprocity and Deviance: An Empirical Extension of Gouldner and Rosenfeld Based on Wills of Providence, 1985." *Sociological Quarterly* 41:265–275.

Sevak, Purvi, and Lina Walker. 2007. *The Responsiveness of Private Savings to Medicaid Long-Term Care Policies.* Ann Arbor: Michigan Retirement Research Center.

Shammas, Carole, Marylynn Salmon, and Michel Dahlin. 1997. *Inheritance in America: From Colonial Times to the Present.* Galveston, TX: Frontier Press.

Shapiro, Thomas M. 2003. *The Hidden Cost of Being African American: How Wealth Perpetuates Inequality.* New York: Oxford University Press.

Short, Pamela, Peter Kemper, Llewellyn J. Cornelius, and Daniel C. Walden. 1992. "Public and Private Responsibility for Financing Nursing Home Care: The Effect of Medicaid Spend-down." *Milbank Quarterly* 70:277–298.

Silverstein, Merril, Stephen J. Conroy, Haitao Wang, Roseann Giarrusso, and Vern L. Bengtson. 2002. "Reciprocity in Parent-Child Relations over the Adult Life Course." *Journal of Gerontology: Social Sciences* 57B: S3–S13.

Silverstein, Merril, Leora Lawton, and Vern L. Bengtson. 1994. "Types of Relations between Parents and Adult Children." Pp. 43–76 in *Intergenerational Linkages: Hidden Connections in American Society.* New York: Springer.

Silverstein, Merril, and Linda J. Waite. 1993. "Are Blacks More Likely than Whites to Receive and Provide Social Support in Middle and Old Age? Yes, No, and Maybe So." *Journal of Gerontology* 48: S212–S222.

Simmel, Georg. 1964. Edited and translated by Kurt H. Wolff. *The Sociology of Georg Simmel.* New York: Free Press.

Smeeding, Timothy, Lee Rainwater, and Michael Higgins, eds. 1990. *Poverty, Inequality and Income Distribution in Comparative Perspective: The Luxembourg Income Study.* London: Harvester Wheatsheaf; Washington, DC: Urban Institute Press.

Smeeding, Timothy M., and James P. Smith. 1998. *The Economic Status of the Elderly on the Eve of Social Security Reform*. Washington, DC: Progressive Policy Institute.

Smerglia, Virginia L., Gary T. Deimling, and Charles M. Barresi. 1988. "Black/White Family Comparisons in Helping and Decision-Making Networks of Impaired Elderly." *Family Relations* 37:305–309.

Smith, Denise. 2003. "The Older Population in the United States: March 2002." *Current Population Reports* P20-546:1–6.

Smith, James P. 1997. "Wealth Inequality among Older Americans." *Journal of Gerontology: Social Sciences* 52B (special issue): 74–81.

Smith, James P., and Raynard Kington. 1997. "Socioeconomic Status and Racial and Ethnic Differences in Functional Status Associated with Chronic Diseases," *American Journal of Public Health* 87:805–810.

Smith, Kristin. 2002. "Who's Minding the Kids? Child Care Arrangements: Spring 1997." *Current Population Reports* P70-86:1–20.

Social Security Administration. 2005. *Annual Statistical Supplement, 2004*. Washington, DC: Government Printing Office.

———. 2006. "2007 Social Security Changes." Retrieved April 22, 2007, from www.ssa.gov/pressoffice/colafacts.htm.

Sokolovsky, Jay. 1985. "Ethnicity, Culture and Aging: Do Differences Really Make a Difference?" *Journal of Applied Gerontology* 4:6–17.

Soldo, Beth J., and Vicky A. Freedman. 1994. "Care of the Elderly: Division of Labor among the Family, Market, and State." Pp. 195–216 in *Demography of Aging*, edited by L. G. Martin and S. H. Preston. Washington, DC: National Academy Press.

Soldo, Beth J., Michael D. Hurd, Willard L. Rodgers, and Robert B. Wallace. 1997. "Asset and Health Dynamics among the Oldest-Old (AHEAD): An Overview of the AHEAD Study." *Journal of Gerontology: Social Sciences* 52B (special): 1–20.

Soldo, Beth J., Douglas A. Wolf, and Emily M. Agree. 1990. "Family, Household, and Care Arrangements of Frail Older Women." *Journal of Gerontology: Social Sciences* 45: S238–S249.

Speas, Kathy, and Beth Obenshain. 1995. *Images of Aging in America*. Washington, DC: AARP.

Spillman, B., and James Lubitz. 2000. "The Effect of Longevity on Spending for Acute and Long-Term Care." *Massachusetts Medical Society* 342:1409–1415.

Steelman, Lala Carr, and Brian Powell. 1989. "Acquiring Capital for College: The Constraints of Family Configuration." *American Sociological Review* 54:844–855.

———. 1991. "Sponsoring the Next Generation: Parental Willingness to Pay for Higher Education." *American Journal of Sociology* 96:1505–1529.

Stephenson, Mary. 1996. *Estate Planning: Writing Wills in Maryland*. College Park: University of Maryland. From www.agnr.umd.edu/MCE/Publications/Publication .cfm? ID=30.

Stoeckle, Mary L., Jane E. Doorley, and Rosanna M. McArdle. 1998. "Identifying Compliance with End-of-life Care Decision Protocols." *Dimensions of Critical Care Nursing* 17 (6): 314–321.

Stoller, Eleanor Palo. 1983. "Parental Caregiving by Adult Children." *Journal of Marriage and the Family* 45:851–858.

Stone, Robyn I. 2000. *Long-term Care for the Elderly with Disabilities: Current Policy, Emerging Trends, and Implications for the Twenty-First Century*. Milbank Memorial Fund. Retrieved July 7, 2004, from www.milbank.org/reports/0008stone/.

Strawbridge, William J., and Margaret I. Wallhagen. 1992. "Is All in the Family Always Best?" *Journal of Aging Studies* 6:81–92.

Stum, Marlene S. 1998. "The Meaning and Experience of Spending Down to Medicaid in Later Life." *Advancing Consumer Interest* 10:23–33.

Suitor, J. Jill, and Karl Pillemer. 1987. "The Presence of Adult Children: A Source of Stress for Elderly Couples' Marriages?" *Journal of Marriage and the Family* 49:717–725.

Sullivan, T. A., Elizabeth Warren, Jay L. Westbrook. 1999. *As We Forgive Our Debtors: Bankruptcy and Consumer Credit in America*. Washington, DC: Beard Books.

Sussman, Marvin B. 1970. *The Family and Inheritance*. New York: Russell Sage Foundation.

Sussman, Marvin B., Judith N. Cates, and David T. Smith. 1990. *The Family and Inheritance*. New York: Russell Sage Foundation.

Sweet, James A., and Larry L. Bumpass. 1987. *American Families and Households*. New York: Russell Sage Foundation.

Talbott, Maria M. 1990. "The Negative Side of the Relationship between Older Widows and Their Adult Children: The Mothers' Perspective." *The Gerontologist* 30:595–603.

Taylor, Robert J. 1985. "The Extended Family as a Source of Support to Elderly Blacks." *The Gerontologist* 25:488–495.

———. 1986. "Receipt of Support from Family among Black Americans: Demographic and Familial Differences." *Journal of Marriage and the Family* 48:67–77.

Taylor, Robert J., and L. M. Chatters. 1986. "Patterns of Informal Support to Elderly Black Adults: Family, Friends, and Church Members." *Social Work* (November–December): 432–437.

Teitler, Michael F. 1986. "Contingency Planning for Incapacity: Powers of Attorney, Revocable Trusts, Health Care Decisions and Living Wills, Committees and Conservators, and 'Informal Arrangements.'" New York: Practising Law Institute, Estate Planning and Administration (Order No. D4-5186).

Texas Administrative Code. 1995. Medicaid Estate Recovery Program, Title 1, Part 15, Chapter 373.

Texas Office of the Secretary of State. 2004. "Medicaid Eligibility: *Texas Administrative Code*, Title 40, Part 1, Chapter 15." Retrieved January 3, 2005, from info.sos.state.tx.us/pls/pub/readtact.ViewTAC?tac_view=4&ti=40&pt=1&ch=15.

Texas Probate Code. Classification of Claims Against Estates of Decedents, Section 322.

Thompson, Linda, and Alexis J. Walker. 1984. "Mothers and Daughters: Aid Patterns and Attachment." *Journal of Marriage and the Family* 46:313–322.

Thornton, Arland, Terri L. Orbuch, and William G. Axinn. 1995. "Parent-Child Relationships during the Transition to Adulthood." *Journal of Family Issues* 16:538–564.

Tienda, M., and F. Mitchell. 2006. *Hispanics and the Future of America*. New York: National Academy Press.

Tocqueville, Alexis de. 1966. *Democracy in America*, edited by J. P. Mayer and Max Lerner. New York: Harper and Row.

———. 1990. *Democracy in America*. Volume 1, chapter 3. New York: Vintage.

Torres-Gil, Fernando M. 1992. *The New Aging: Politics and Change in America*. Westport, CT: Auburn House.

Treas, Judith. 1977. "Family Support Systems for the Aged: Some Social and Demographic Considerations." *The Gerontologist* 17:486–491.

Troll, Lillian E. 1971. "The Family of Later Life: A Decade Review." *Journal of Marriage and the Family* 33:263–290.

Trout, Peggy S. 1997. *Adequacy and Equity of Social Security. Report of 1994–1996 Advisory Council on Social Security*, vol. 2, *Findings and Recommendations*. Washington, DC: Government Printing Office.

Tucker, Robert C., ed. 1978. *The Marx-Engels Reader*. New York: W. W. Norton.

Uhlenberg, Peter. 1992. "Population Aging and Social Policy." *Annual Review of Sociology* 18:449–474.

Umberson, Debra. 1992. "Relationships between Adult Children and Their Parents: Psychological Consequences for Both Generations." *Journal of Marriage and the Family* 54:664–674.

———. 2006. "Parents, Adult Children, and Immortality." *Contexts* 5:48–53.

U.S. Census Bureau. 2002. "Poverty in the United States: 2001." *Current Population Reports*, P60-219. Washington, DC: Government Printing Office.

———. 2003. "Hispanic Population Reaches All-Time High of 38.8 Million, New Census Bureau Estimates Show." *U.S. Census Bureau News*, June 18. Washington, DC: U.S. Department of Commerce. Retrieved January 3, 2005, from www.census.gov/Press-Release/www/releases/archives/hispanic_origin_population/001130.html.

———. 2004a. "Nation Adds 3 Million People in Last Year; Nevada Again Fastest-Growing State." *U.S. Census Bureau News*, December 22. Washington, DC: U.S. Department of Commerce. Retrieved January 3, 2005, from www.census.gov/Press-Release/www/releases/archives/population/003153.html.

———. 2004b. "Resident Population by Race, Hispanic or Latino Origin, and State: 2003." *Statistical Abstracts of the United States*. Table No. 21. Washington, DC: Government Printing Office.

———. 2006. "Expectation of Life and Expected Deaths, by Race, Sex, and Age: 2003." *The 2007 Statistical Abstract*. Washington, DC: Government Printing Office.

U.S. Department of Health and Human Services. 2007. *Paying for Long-term Care: Overview*. National Clearinghouse for Long-term Care Information. www.longtermcare.gov/LTC/Main_Site/Paying_LTC/Costs_Of_Care/Costs_Of_Care.aspx.

U.S. Department of Health and Human Services, Office of Disability, Aging and Long-Term Care Policy. 2005. *Medicaid Estate Recovery*. Washington, DC: Office of the Assistant Secretary for Planning and Evaluation. Retrieved April 25, 2007, aspe.hhs.gov/daltcp/reports/estaterec.htm.

U.S. Department of Labor. 2000. *The Needs of Families and Employers: The Family and Medical Leave Surveys*. Washington, DC: Government Printing Office.

U.S. Office of Personnel Management. 2006. "About the Program: Federal Long-term Care Insurance (Public Law 106-265)." Retrieved January 3, 2007, from www.ltcfeds.com/about/106-265.pdf.

Walker, Alexis J., and Linda Thompson. 1983. "Intimacy and Intergenerational Aid and Contact Among Mothers and Daughters." *Journal of Marriage and the Family* 45:841–849.

Wallace, Stephen P., Veronica F. Gutierrez. 2005. "Equity of Access to Health Care for Older Adults in Four Major Latin American Cities." *Pan American Journal of Public Health* 17:394–409.

Walsh, Mary Williams. 2005. "U.S. Agrees to Take Over Four Pension Plans at United." *New York Times*, April 23. Retrieved May 3, 2005, from select.nytimes.com/search/restricted/article?res=FB061EF83F550C708EDDAD0894DD404482.

Ward, Russell A., and Glenna Spitze. 1992. "Consequences of Parent-Adult Child Coresidence." *Journal of Family Issues* 13:553–572.

Weinick, Robin M. 1995. "Sharing a Home: The Experiences of American Women and Their Parents over the Twentieth Century." *Demography* 32:281–297.

Weisman, Jonathan. 2003. "Despite Win, Estate-Tax Momentum Decreasing." *Daily Iowan*, June 19. Retrieved July 7, 2004, from www.dailyiowan.com/news/2003/06/19/Nation/Despite.Win.EstateTax.Momentum.Decreasing-439884.shtml.

White, Lynn, Alan Booth, and John N. Edwards. 1992. "The Effect of Parental Divorce and Remarriage on Parental Support for Adult Children." *Journal of Family Issues* 13 (2) (special issue): 234–250.

White-Means, Shelley I., and Michael C. Thornton. 1990. "Ethnic Differences in the Production of Informal Home Health Care." *The Gerontologist* 30:758–768.

Wiener, Joshua M. 1996. "Public Policies on Medicaid Asset Transfer and Estate Recovery: How Much Money to Be Saved?" *Generations* 20:72–76.

Wiener, Joshua M., and David G. Stevenson. 1997. "Long-term Care for the Elderly and State Health Policy." *New Federalism: Issues and Options for States*. Series Number A-17. Washington, DC: Urban Institute.

Wilhelm, Mark O. 1996. "Bequest Behavior and the Effect of Heirs' Earnings: Testing the Altruistic Model of Bequests." *American Economic Review* (September): 874–892.

Williamson, John B., Diane Watts-Roy, and Eric R. Kingson, eds. 1999. *The Generational Equity Debate*. New York: Columbia University Press.

Wilmoth, Janet M., and Gregor Koso. 2002. "Does Marital History Matter? The Effect of Marital Status on Wealth Outcomes among Pre-retirement-age Adults." *Journal of Marriage and Family* 64:254–268.

Wilson, Barbara Foley, and Sally Cunningham Clarke. 1992. "Remarriages: A Demographic Profile." *Journal of Family Issues* 13:123–141.

Wilson, William J. 1996. *When Work Disappears: The World of the Urban Poor*. New York: Knopf.

Winick, Charles. 1972. *Dictionary of Anthropology*. Totowa, NJ: Littlefield.

Wise, David A., ed. 1996. *Advances in the Economics of Aging*. Chicago: University of Chicago Press.

Wolf, Douglas A. 2001. "Everything Is Relatives: Intergenerational Relationships, Public Policies, and Eldercare." Invited paper presented at the Aging in the Americas Policy Roundtable, 2001, University of Texas at Austin.

Wolff, Edward N. 1998. "Recent Trends in the Size Distribution of Household Wealth." *Journal of Economic Perspectives* 12:131–150.

———. 2003. "The Impact of Gifts and Bequests on the Distribution of Wealth." Pp. 345–375 in *Death and Dollars*, edited by A. H. Munnell and A. Sundén. Washington, DC: Brookings Institution.

Wong, Rebeca, Chiara Capoferro, and Beth J. Soldo. 1999. "Financial Assistance from Middle-Aged Couples to Parents and Children: Racial-Ethnic Differences." *Journal of Gerontology: Social Sciences* 54B: S145–S153.

Wong, Rebeca, Kathy Kitayama, and Beth J. Soldo. 1999. "Ethnic Differences in Time Transfers from Adult Children to Elderly Parents: Unobserved Heterogeneity across Families." *Research on Aging* 21:144–175.

World Bank. 1994. *Averting the Old Age Crisis*. Washington, DC: World Bank.

Wray, Linda A., and Duane F. Alwin. 2005. "A Life-Span Developmental Perspective on Social Status and Health," *Journal of Gerontology: Social Sciences* 60 (special issue): 7–14.

Young, Rosalie F., and Eva Kahana. 1985. "The Context of Caregiving and Well-Being Outcomes among African and Caucasian Americans." *The Gerontologist* 35:225–232.

Zelizer, Viviana A. 1996. "Payments and Social Ties." *Sociological Forum* 11:481–495.

———. 1997. *The Social Meaning of Money*. Princeton, NJ: Princeton University Press.

———. 1998. "How People Talk About Money." *American Behavioral Scientist* 41 (special issue): 1373–1383.

Zick, Catherine D., and Ken R. Smith. 1991. "Patterns of Economic Change surrounding the Death of a Spouse." *Journal of Gerontology: Social Sciences* 46: S310–S320.

Index